Strategic Implications of HIV/AIDS

Stefan Elbe

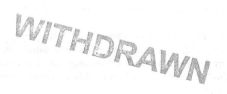
ADELPHI PAPER 357

9181151

Oxford University Press, Great Clarendon Street, Oxford OX2 6DP
Oxford New York
Athens Auckland Bangkok Bombay Calcutta Cape Town
Dar es Salaam Delhi Florence Hong Kong Istanbul Karachi
Kuala Lumpur Madras Madrid Melbourne Mexico City Nairobi
Paris Taipei Tokyo Toronto
and associated companies in Ibadan

Oxford is a trade mark of Oxford University Press

Published in the United States
by Oxford University Press Inc., New York

© The International Institute for Strategic Studies 2003

First published June 2003 by **Oxford University Press** for
The International Institute for Strategic Studies
Arundel House, 13–15 Arundel Street, Temple Place, London WC2R 3DX
www.iiss.org

Director John Chipman
Editor Tim Huxley
Copy Editor Matthew Foley
Production Simon Nevitt/Shirley Nicholls

British Library Cataloguing in Publication Data
Data available

Library of Congress Cataloguing in Publication Data

ISBN 0-19-852912-0
ISSN 0567-932x

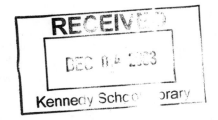

Contents

Tables

Introduction

The scourge of war still constitutes the greatest threat to human existence and well-being as we cross the threshold of the twenty-first century. So, at least, argues the distinguished military historian John Keegan. In Keegan's view, war has overtaken 'disease and famine in the hierarchy of threats this world offers to human life, liberty and happiness'.[1] This paper challenges this view in light of the 25 million people thought to have died from AIDS-related illnesses over the past two decades, and the additional 42m people estimated to be living with HIV/AIDS around the world.[2] In many countries in Sub-Saharan Africa, HIV has infected between a tenth and a third of the adult population; AIDS has outgrown war as the leading cause of death in Africa by a factor of ten.[3] Many other regions of strategic significance may be similarly affected in years to come. At least in numerical terms, AIDS is becoming a far greater threat to human existence than armed conflict; in the next decade alone, the pandemic is expected to kill more human beings than all the combatants killed in the First World War, the Second World War, the Korean War and the Vietnam War combined. While this is not to diminish the continued relevance of more conventional strategic issues, it will be necessary to acknowledge new challenges – including those emanating from outside the military domain.

First and foremost, the AIDS pandemic is undoubtedly a humanitarian and human security issue in the sense of bringing widespread suffering, impoverishment and death to millions of people around the world. This immense humanitarian dimension of the illness must ultimately guide our thinking about it, and inform the international response to it. Yet this should not lead policymakers to overlook the fact that the AIDS pandemic also has an important strategic dimension. Unlike many other illnesses, HIV/AIDS does not spread exclusively amongst the poor, the very young or the old; in many countries, it is also cutting through political, military and economic elites – often affecting them at their most productive age. This aspect of the illness, compounded by the magnitude of the pandemic, means that in some countries HIV/AIDS is beginning to intersect with more traditional strategic concerns surrounding the deployment of armed force in international relations. Around the globe, members of the security sector are profoundly affected by, and important actors in, this wider AIDS pandemic. Consequently, the security sector will have to engage in more sustained efforts to anticipate the possible strategic ramifications of the illness in the years ahead, while simultaneously reflecting on how it can make a responsible contribution to international efforts to reduce the transmission of HIV. In the case of HIV/AIDS, sound strategic planning and humanitarian concerns can overlap considerably.

The strategic dimension of the AIDS pandemic is currently emerging along two distinct but closely-related axes. The first revolves around the disproportionately high prevalence of HIV/AIDS in many countries' armed forces. Several militaries in Africa and Asia are thought to have prevalence rates significantly higher than those of their countries' civilian adult population. In some African militaries, prevalence rates are estimated to be as high as 40% or 60%, raising serious questions about combat readiness and effectiveness. Some of these armed forces regularly participate in peacekeeping operations, contributing to the spread of HIV in the areas in which they are deployed and damaging the international reputation of these operations. The first question that emerges in relation to the long-term strategic implications of the AIDS pandemic, therefore, is what impact HIV and AIDS have on the armed forces in those countries where prevalence rates are high, and the domestic and international strategic ramifications of this in the long term.

The second strategic dimension of the AIDS pandemic is its potential to act as a politically destabilising force. The fact that, in many countries, HIV/AIDS is spreading amongst the elite and middle classes is giving rise to concerns about the long-term effects on the political, economic and social stability of states with high prevalence rates. Some combatants in recent armed conflicts may even have hoped that the illness would have precisely such destabilising effects. In Rwanda, for example, survivors of the genocide have claimed that HIV, passed through rape, was used as a weapon of war, aimed at subjecting victims to economic hardship, psychological stress, illness and, ultimately, death.[4] Destabilising developments in one country could potentially induce more widespread regional instability, with concomitantly larger strategic ramifications not only for those societies directly affected, but also for actors with interests in these regions, and for those charged with maintaining international peace and security. It will therefore be necessary to reflect in greater detail on the extent to which the AIDS pandemic could also contribute to political instability, and, if so, where it might do so.

Despite the importance of these emerging questions, the debate about the strategic implications of HIV/AIDS remains in its infancy. It is also marked by two shortcomings. First, opinion amongst analysts and policymakers is polarised between those trying to portray HIV/AIDS as a strategic issue of catastrophic dimensions, and the more traditional strategic establishment that remains reserved about this designation, finding the strategic dimension of AIDS to be much less evident than suggested. While HIV/AIDS is clearly a humanitarian issue of almost unimaginable magnitude, there is controversy about the analytically more challenging and sensitive question of whether it also amounts to a strategic issue in the conventional sense of potentially contributing to the outbreak of armed conflict. Much of this disagreement has not yet been rehearsed in public, and critics of the core proposition that HIV/AIDS is a strategic issue have largely chosen to remain silent, hoping, perhaps, that the question will gradually disappear from the strategic agenda.[5] Nevertheless, this sharp divergence in opinion points to the need for further research on the relationship between HIV/AIDS and the deployment of armed force.

The second shortcoming of the debate on the strategic dimension of HIV/AIDS is a lack of appreciation of its complexity. Neither side of the debate has yet been able to adequately incorporate the subtle nature of many of the impacts of HIV/AIDS on the deployment of armed force. How exactly the strategic implications of HIV/AIDS might unfold is only poorly understood at present.[6] Even if, as is increasingly suggested, HIV/AIDS will have long-term strategic ramifications for the use of military force in the international system, current arguments will undoubtedly have to be further refined and spelled out in greater detail in order to be convincing on a broader basis and to stimulate wider public debate.

This paper thus raises five key questions regarding the long-term strategic dimensions of the AIDS pandemic.

1. What is the current scope of the AIDS pandemic in civilian and military populations?
2. What is the impact of HIV/AIDS on the armed forces in countries with high prevalence rates?
3. How does HIV/AIDS affect international peacekeeping operations?
4. What is the impact of the AIDS pandemic on the political stability of the worst-affected states?
5. How should the security sector respond to the strategic dimensions of AIDS?

This paper constitutes an initial, exploratory 'think piece'. It argues that the starting-point for a mature and responsible debate on the strategic dimensions of HIV/AIDS has to be a candid admission that an insufficient amount of reliable information is available in the public domain to answer these questions with certainty. The absence of reliable data is a major impediment to fully understanding the strategic dimension of the illness. It will also be necessary to acknowledge that the strategic dimensions of HIV/AIDS are unlikely to emerge in a uniform and generic fashion around the world. There are likely to be important variations within the worst-affected regions, and important questions remain about the extent to which other regions of the world will emulate the plight of Sub-Saharan Africa. This suggests the need for a two-fold approach: first, it will be necessary to identify the key variables that are likely to determine the strategic dimensions of HIV/AIDS in general. This is the aim of this paper. Second, future research will need to focus on country-specific studies that analyse and assess these variables on a case-by-case basis.

Most of the preliminary evidence indicates that the AIDS pandemic is likely to have an important strategic dimension, presenting new and serious challenges to the stability of governments controlling the use of armed force in international relations, as well as for the militaries responsible for implementing any decision to deploy such force. This dimension is already emerging in Africa and to some extent in Asia, and its magnitude is likely to grow considerably as mortality rates increase. At the same time, this strategic dimension of HIV/AIDS does not have to be as catastrophic as the current humanitarian crisis, if addressed now on the basis of a broader and concerted international approach, to which the security sector can make a crucial contribution.

Chapter 1

Health, strategy and HIV/AIDS

Widespread infectious illnesses have long had a profound influence on the course of human events. Historically, they have facilitated important reconfigurations of political power and have even contributed to the demise of entire societies. In the ancient world, the plague of Athens hastened the collapse of the Athenian empire.[1] In fourteenth-century Europe, bubonic plague killed around 24m people, accelerating a host of complex social, economic and political changes. In the sixteenth century, diseases played a crucial role in establishing European hegemony over many other parts of the globe, constituting one of the most important factors in the demise of the Aztec and Inca empires, for example, as Europeans brought with them a variety of diseases to which the Amerindians had little or no resistance.[2]

Widespread illnesses have historically also had narrower strategic implications through their disproportionately high impact on soldiers and combatants, and thus also on battle outcomes. Writing two years prior to the outbreak of the Second World War, American microbiologist Hans Zinsser advanced the provocative thesis that soldiers have only rarely won wars; rather, they 'more often mop up after the barrage of epidemics. And typhus, with its brothers and sisters, – plague, cholera, typhoid, dysentery – has decided more campaigns than Caesar, Hannibal, Napoleon, and all the inspector generals of history. The epidemics get the blame for defeat, the generals the credit for victory'.[3] Disease has indeed played a crucial, if not decisive, role in some important battles. Trachoma among his troops jeopardised Napoleon's entire expedition in Egypt, for example, while his advance into Syria was frustrated by an outbreak of bubonic plague as he was trying to seize St. John of Acre, only 90 miles from Jerusalem.[4] With characteristic hubris, Napoleon would later reflect on St. Helena that, had St. John of Acre fallen, 'I would have changed the face of the world'.[5]

Although the West has experienced both the broader and narrower strategic importance of widespread illnesses in the past, memory of this legacy largely died in the latter half of the twentieth century. Following the First World War, a crucial change occurred in the West's threat perceptions, as the threat posed by large-scale industrial warfare began to supersede the perceived relevance of widespread diseases. In the aftermath of the Second World War, especially, the West saw the greatest threat to human existence as residing in the outbreak of industrial and even nuclear war. Important advances in medicine reinforced this impression. Strategic thinking evolved in a way that reflected this important change, and began to aim at achieving a better understanding of the dynamics of large-scale warfare and nuclear deterrence. This understanding of strategy may have been an appropriate response to the geopolitics of the twentieth century, but it also makes it more difficult for Western strategists today to entertain the possibility that widespread illnesses might acquire renewed strategic significance. Outside the West, by contrast, it is much less difficult to see this connection, as infectious diseases including HIV/AIDS assume proportions that are clearly comparable to earlier epidemics in terms of numbers of people affected.

HIV prevalence in civilian populations

The magnitude of the AIDS pandemic is clearly immense, yet determining its exact extent is fraught with complex difficulties. Some of the most comprehensive data has been compiled jointly by the World Health Organisation (WHO) and UNAIDS. Even these figures are, however, estimates only, and are subject to considerable logistical problems and political pressures, many of them currently beyond the control of UNAIDS. Global figures issued by UNAIDS in December 2002 estimate that 42m people are living with HIV or AIDS. Of these, 38.6m are thought to be adults (between 15 and 49 years old), and 3.2m children (under 15 years of age). UNAIDS estimates that around 25m people have died from AIDS-related illnesses. In 2002, an estimated 3.1m people died of AIDS-related illnesses, and there were 5m new HIV transmissions. These figures indicate that the AIDS pandemic is, at least in numerical terms, amongst the worst ever to have confronted mankind; in the first decade of the twenty-first century, its victims could exceed those of the Spanish Influenza epidemic of 1918–19, which is estimated to have caused between 25m and 40m deaths worldwide.[6] It will also exceed the number of victims of the bubonic plague in Europe.

Every region of the world currently has a significant number of people living with HIV and AIDS. This means that the illness is best thought of as a pandemic, rather than merely as an epidemic. Although Sub-Saharan Africa is presently worst-affected, epidemiological indicators show that the illness is spreading quickly in Asia, the Indian subcontinent and the Caribbean, as well as in Russia and Eastern Europe. Table 1 gives current UNAIDS estimates for the regional distribution of HIV/AIDS at the end of 2002.

Table 1: The Regional Distribution of HIV/AIDS, end-2002

Region	Adults and Children Living with HIV	Adults and Children Newly Infected with HIV
Sub-Saharan Africa	29,400,000	3,500,000
North Africa and the Middle East	550,000	83,000
South and South-East Asia	6,000,000	700,000
East Asia and the Pacific	1,200,000	270,000
Latin America	1,500,000	150,000
The Caribbean	440,000	60,000
Eastern Europe and Central Asia	1,200,000	250,000
Western Europe	570,000	30,000
North America	980,000	45,000
Australia and New Zealand	15,000	500
Total	**42,000,000**	**5,000,000**

Source: 'AIDS Epidemic Update', UNAIDS, Geneva, December 2002

Africa has been hit particularly hard, and is the area of greatest importance in considering the probable broader strategic implications of HIV/AIDS. This is where the strategic ramifications of HIV/AIDS are most likely to emerge first. Table 2 shows the adult HIV prevalence rates for several African countries, estimated by UNAIDS in December 2001. There are important variations between different regions. In Kenya, for example, prevalence rates have reached 15% of the adult population; in western Africa, at least five countries are close to or above the 5% prevalence mark, after which it becomes increasingly difficult to control the spread of the illness in the general population. In southern Africa, where the situation is worst, countries such as Zimbabwe and Botswana are thought to have prevalence rates in excess of one-third of the adult population, with many more ranging between 10% and 20%.

Table 2: HIV Prevalence in Africa

Country	Percentage of Adult Population (15–49) Infected with HIV or Suffering from AIDS	Number of Adults and Children Living with HIV/AIDS
Botswana	38.8%	330,000
Swaziland	33.4%	170,000
Zimbabwe	33.7%	2,300,000
Lesotho	31.0%	360,000
Zambia	21.5%	1,200,000
South Africa	20.1%	5,000,000
Namibia	22.5%	230,000
Malawi	15.0%	850,000
Kenya	15.0%	2,500,000
Central African Republic	12.9%	250,000
Mozambique	13.0%	1,100,000
Rwanda	8.9%	500,000

Source: 'Report on the Global HIV/AIDS Epidemic', UNAIDS, July 2002

Data is also beginning to emerge from Asia. In Asia and the Pacific, 7.1m people are thought to be living with HIV. Cambodia, Myanmar and Thailand all have prevalence rates exceeding 1% of those between the age of 15 and 49. One percent of the national adult population may not seem like a very significant figure in strategic terms, but it is worth recalling that in South Africa as recently as 1990 less than one percent of pregnant women attending antenatal clinics tested HIV-positive. Only a decade later, South Africa had officially become the country with the largest number of people living with HIV/AIDS in the world. If not adequately addressed, serious epidemics could also emerge in Asia over the course of the next decade, especially in populous countries such as China and India. China has already registered HIV cases in all of its 31 provinces, with an estimated half a million to a million of its people living with HIV.[7] The Chinese Ministry of Health projects that there will be up to 10m cases by 2010 if effective precautions are not taken.[8] Official figures in India put the number of HIV-positive people at 3.97m, though some unofficial estimates place the figure closer to 5m.[9] Both India and China, home to a third of the world's population and of major strategic significance, are thus on the verge of more widespread epidemics; it is thought that the region as a whole might surpass Africa in the absolute number of infections by 2010.

Growth rates in Russia and Eastern Europe are presently the highest in the world, with an estimated 250,000 new infections in 2001, bringing to one million the regional total of people thought to be living with HIV. At the end of 2001, Ukraine alone had an estimated 250,000 infected people, making this the worst epidemic in Europe, with 1% of adults HIV-positive.[10] In Latin America and the Caribbean, 12 countries have estimated adult prevalence rates of more than 1%.[11] These figures suggest that strategic analysts in Western countries, where prevalence rates remain relatively low, cannot afford to underestimate the scale of the pandemic. Nor can they view HIV/AIDS exclusively as an African issue.

HIV prevalence in military populations

Data on HIV prevalence in armed forces around the world is even harder to obtain than epidemiological data about rates amongst general populations, and consequently is very patchy. Armed forces, particularly ones in which prevalence rates are thought to be high, are usually hesitant to make such information public, if it exists at all, because of the potential vulnerabilities it would highlight. The available data is, however, sufficient as a broad indicator of trends. One important conclusion it points to is that HIV prevalence in many armed forces appears to be higher than in the surrounding civilian population. UNAIDS studies indicate that the peacetime prevalence rate of sexually-transmitted diseases amongst military populations is generally between two and five times higher than it is among the national adult population.[12] In a study declassified in January 2000, the National Intelligence Council (NIC) in the US estimated HIV prevalence rates in selected military populations in Sub-Saharan Africa in 1999. These figures, shown in Table 3, were supplied by the Armed Forces Medical Intelligence Center, part of the US Defense Intelligence Agency.

Table 3: Estimated HIV Prevalence Rates in Selected Military and Civilian Populations in Africa, 1999

Country	Military Population	Adult Population
Angola	40–60%	2.78%
Congo (Brazzaville)	10–25%	6.43%
Côte d'Ivoire	10-20%	10.76%
Democratic Republic of Congo	40–60%	5.07%
Eritrea	10%	2.87%
Nigeria	10–20%	5.06%
Tanzania	15–30%	8.09%

Sources: 'The Global Infectious Disease Threat and Its Implications for the United States', report of the National Intelligence Council, NIE 99-17D, January 2000; 'The Global Strategy Framework on HIV/AIDS', UNAIDS, June 2001, p. 3; 'Report on the Global HIV/AIDS Epidemic', UNAIDS, July 2002

According to these figures, several armed forces in Sub-Saharan Africa have HIV prevalence rates of around 10% to 20%, with some as high as 60%.[13] Yet it is not clear from the NIC report how these figures were obtained, or how robust these estimates are; UNAIDS, for example, has reported HIV prevalence amongst the Tanzanian uniformed services to be between 15% and 16%.[14] A study by Lindy Heinecken, of the Centre for Military Studies (CEMIS) at the South African Military Academy, gives rates similar to the NIC report, based on a defence intelligence assessment carried out by the South African government. These figures are given in Table 4.

Table 4: HIV Prevalence Rates in Selected African Militaries

Country	HIV Prevalence	Date of Estimate
Angola	50%	1999
Botswana	33%	1999
DRC	50%	1999
Lesotho	40%	1999
Malawi	50%	1999
Namibia	16%	1999
South Africa	15–20%	2000
Swaziland	48%	1997
Zambia	60%	1998
Zimbabwe	55%	1999

Source: Lindy Heinecken, 'Living in Terror: The Looming Security Threat to Southern Africa', *African Security Review*, vol. 10, no. 4, 2001, p. 11

In South Africa, official rates for military infection of between 17% and 23% do not far exceed corresponding civilian rates, but these figures are thought by some analysts to be unreliable given that soldiers are only tested on deployment, and the majority of the force is currently not deployable.[15] Earlier unofficial estimates speculated that the figure may even be between 40% and 60% of soldiers. Leaked figures reveal that, in some areas, 60% to 70% of soldiers might be infected with HIV.[16] In one military police base in northern KwaZulu-Natal, the figure was as high as 90%, with 30 out of 33 of those evaluated testing positive.[17] Units based around Pietermaritzburg and the South Africa–Mozambique border may have prevalence rates upwards of 70%.[18] In Namibia, unofficial estimates suggest that one-third of the armed forces was infected as of 2001.[19] Studies have also been carried out on specific sections of particular armed forces. In Sierra Leone, for example, more than 21% of 1,099 candidates screened in a recruitment process in 2001 were HIV-positive.[20] Older figures are available for several other African countries.[21]

In Asia, a newspaper report in 1998 controversially claimed that 6,000 members of the Indian army had tested HIV-positive, while HIV prevalence amongst the Cambodian military reportedly ranges between 6% and 17%.[22] The situation is particularly serious in the province of Koh Kong bordering Thailand, where up to 30% of the armed forces, and 10.5% of the police force, are reported to have tested positive for HIV in 1995.[23] Subsequent studies carried out in the province indicated a 10% prevalence rate among military personnel in 1997 and a 25.8% prevalence rate among the police force in 1998.[24] The prevalence rate among recruits from the north of the country is 4%.[25] This had been as high as 12.5% in 1991, before the Thai military took steps to reduce it, such as promoting condom use.[26] In Ba Ria Vung Tau province in southern Vietnam, prevalence rates among young army recruits in early 2002 were reported to be 4.5%, while in Myanmar a study carried out in Mandalay and Yangon in 1997 showed a 5% prevalence rate in the 20–24 age group.[27] In these countries, HIV prevalence amongst the armed forces tends to exceed that of the civilian population. In the first half of 2000, there were 260 new reported cases of HIV infection among Russian troops, though rates could well be ten times higher.[28] In Latin America, Brazil reported in 1996 that 1,396 military personnel were living with HIV out of a total of roughly 200,000 troops.[29] In Haiti, the prevalence rate among the military in 1995 was reported to be around 10%.[30]

One of the reasons for higher prevalence rates among armed forces when compared to civilian populations is that soldiers' duties require them to be geographically mobile, and to be away from home for extended periods. Troops may engage in casual sexual relations while on tour, and large concentrations of soldiers may attract a high number of sex workers, especially when deployed in areas of material scarcity. Alcohol and other drugs used to cope with the pressures of military existence can further increase the chances of unprotected sexual intercourse, while sexual activity, whether consensual or forced, typically increases in times of conflict.[32] These risk factors can also be exacerbated by military culture. There may also be peer pressure amongst soldiers to engage in sexual activities.[31] In many armed forces, risky behaviour is valorised, and this ethos can carry over into a soldier's sexual relations, influencing crucial decisions about condom use, for instance.

A more indirect reason for these high prevalence rates in the military has to do with the cycle of the illness. Unlike many earlier diseases, which had an immediate impact on affected forces, HIV/AIDS does not lead to a sudden death; rather, after an initial bodily reaction to the infection, it can be a decade before the illness culminates in full-blown AIDS. This means that HIV/AIDS is not an immediate 'war-stopper', and does not instantly bar individual soldiers from carrying out their duties. This enables HIV to spread much further than would be the case if it led to a quick death. It has also allowed military officials to ignore the gravity of the problems raised by HIV.

Western militaries are not immune to these risk factors.[33] Up to 45% of Dutch sailors and marines on a five-month peacekeeping tour in Cambodia in the early 1990s had contact with sex workers, and condom use, the crucial variable, was inconsistent.[34] Between 1989 and 1991, 10% of naval personnel and marines contracted a new sexually-transmitted disease during missions in South America, West Africa and the Mediterranean.[35] According to the French military, French troops are five times more likely to become infected with HIV during an overseas tour of duty, despite repeated warnings of the risks.[36] Between 1985, when tests began, and 2000, the US navy documented 4,680 cases of HIV infection among active-duty sailors and marines.[37] Between 1995 and 1998, condom use among unmarried active-duty personnel across the US military ranged from 37% to 45%.[38]

In many countries, then, the armed forces have high HIV prevalence rates, often exceeding the levels of the civilian population. The armed forces occupationally constitute a high-risk group for the transmission of HIV. These high prevalence rates have clear strategic implications for the deployment of armed force in international relations, and point towards a far more complex domestic and international strategic picture, which is explored in the chapters that follow.

Chapter 2

The impact of HIV/AIDS on armed forces

There is increasing evidence around the world to suggest that HIV/AIDS is posing new challenges for those actors charged with maintaining public order and defending national security. The problem is particularly severe in countries experiencing high HIV prevalence rates, where the security sector is being profoundly affected. In 1996, 34% of all deaths among active-duty military personnel in the Congo were estimated to be AIDS-related.[1] In Zambia and Namibia, AIDS-related illnesses now constitute the leading cause of death among the military and police forces, in some cases accounting for more than half of all deaths in the services.[2] The crucial strategic question, therefore, is not whether HIV/AIDS is having an impact on the armed forces, but rather how, in the worst-affected countries, this impact will manifest itself, and with what overall strategic significance.

The military impact of high HIV prevalence rates

All things being equal, high HIV prevalence rates are likely to diminish the operational efficiency of a country's armed forces. This negative impact would be in line with historical experience. In the Spanish–American War of 1898, for example, virtually every soldier had at one time or another contracted malaria or yellow-fever, decreasing the number of fit personnel available by up to half.[3] Given the long cycle of HIV/AIDS, high prevalence rates are unlikely to have the same immediate impact, especially on those soldiers carrying out combat activities. Nevertheless, HIV/AIDS poses new challenges for a country's armed forces by virtue of its potential impact in four important areas: resources, personnel, morale and relations with the civilian population.

Resource implications

High HIV prevalence rates are likely eventually to entail the training and recruiting of more soldiers to replace personnel who have succumbed to the illness, increasing the amount of human and financial resources expended, particularly if the need is to replace personnel in specialised or technically demanding roles, such as information technology or communications. This is not a one-off cost: it will affect militaries year after year until the pandemic is under better control. As Major James Samba of the Sierra Leone Army (SLA) puts it, there will have to be 'a continuous high level of army recruitment because of this disease'.[4] To this must be added the increased medical costs stemming from caring for the ill and the dying.

Personnel implications

HIV will have a related impact on personnel and staffing. Especially for those countries that seek to exclude people living with HIV from the armed forces, the pandemic means that the available volunteer pool decreases significantly. HIV affects most severely precisely that age group (people between 15 and 24 years of age) from which militaries draw the majority of their soldiers.

In many countries, there will probably be enough young men to meet requirements, but the range of choice will decrease and, where service is not compulsory, there could be an increased demand for these same people from other sectors of society. Moreover, in militaries where HIV testing is compulsory, this may deter potential recruits who are uncertain about their HIV status.[5] The South African National Defence Force (SANDF) has considered launching a compulsory national-service programme in order to maintain operational readiness.[6] In most cases, however, HIV will primarily reduce the number of potential recruits the armed forces have to choose from. This is especially true if applicants to the armed forces perceive this choice of employment as linked to a much greater risk of acquiring HIV/AIDS. HIV/AIDS will also affect the senior level of command,[7] and less experienced soldiers might have to be promoted to fill these positions.

HIV/AIDS can also lead to the loss of highly specialised or technically trained staff. Many of these highly skilled soldiers will not be replaced quickly, easily or cheaply. This will be a problem for those armed forces who have not previously taken these developments into account. These forces may find that it takes them several years to replace such specialised personnel.

Implications for morale and cohesion

HIV/AIDS can also damage morale. Although this area has not been subject to systematic study, knowing that some of their comrades will die slow and painful deaths is unlikely to motivate soldiers, especially if they suspect that they might suffer a similar predicament in the near future. Soldiers may also resent receiving an increased duty load while other troops are ill, or while the position of a dead soldier remains vacant. Operations may run less smoothly as soldiers have to take frequent leave in order to attend the funerals of friends and relatives. According to Namibian Defence Minister Erkki Nghimtina, 'we are seeing frequent burial services, our hospitals record more unfitness for combat activities and sick leaves are on the increase'.[8] In Malawi, considerable time and resources appear to be devoted to arranging and attending the funerals of soldiers.[9] Even if absences can be filled temporarily, or if new recruits can be found to replace ones who have died, the efficient and unhindered functioning and cooperation of units can be compromised if staffed by new personnel, and troops are being deployed together who have not previously enjoyed common operational experience.

The smooth running of military operations may also be compromised as soldiers become aware of the problem of HIV/AIDS, and thus less willing to attend to wounded colleagues for fear of infection. This can become particularly serious in joint and multilateral operations between militaries of different countries and, in the case of serious injury, where there are doubts about the safety of blood supplies. Indeed, the question of how to secure blood supplies during military operations is a growing problem for the efficient execution of such deployments. Again, this is not only a problem in Africa and Asia. NATO has hosted several conferences on blood safety in military and civilian emergencies in light of emerging concerns about the safety of blood reserves.

Implications for civil–military relations

Given the lethal nature of the illness, its social stigma and the important human rights considerations that surround it, HIV/AIDS can cause problems for relations between military and civilian populations. In the US, for example, considerable difficulties arose when an HIV-positive solider stationed at Fort Benning in Georgia had unprotected sexual intercourse with at least eight women between 1995 and 1998.[10] The Rwandan Ministry of Defence has officially recognised the risk that soldiers returning from the DRC may pass HIV on to sexual partners in the civilian population.[11] The military's handling of HIV/AIDS is a wider social issue, and armed forces have had to engage in sustained discussions with civilian society over issues such as the treatment of HIV-positive personnel and the testing of recruits. In Israel, for example, the military's acknowledgement in 1997 that it was routinely testing Jewish soldiers from Ethiopia without their consent provoked political controversy.[12] Some countries have refused entry to US troops if they could not be certified as HIV-negative. In the run-up to the expiry of the Philippines' defence agreement with the US in 1991, activists succeeded in politicising the presence of US forces in the country by accusing them of introducing and spreading HIV/AIDS.[13] The defence agreement was not renewed and, while this issue was certainly not the only reason for this, it could not have helped the US cause.

Beginning to take note

Preliminary evidence suggests that some armed forces are beginning to recognise the new challenges posed by HIV/AIDS. Major-General Matshwenyego Fisher, Chief of Staff of the Botswana Defence Force, has stated that 'AIDS in the military ... is no longer an academic issue; it is a reality that has to be tackled with all the vigour and effort that is commensurate with its ramifications'.[14] According to the Namibian Deputy Minister of Defence, Victor Simunja, HIV/AIDS is 'affecting security and military establishments to the core', while the Rwandan Ministry of Defence considers HIV/AIDS a strategic issue because of its impact on the army and the gendarmerie.[15] According to Heinecken, there are fears within the SANDF that AIDS will decimate the force's middle ranks, as many personnel are expected to die before the age of 35.[16] Half of HIV-positive soldiers in the SANDF are in the 23 to 29 age group, the most deployable section of the force. The SANDF is also concerned that it will not be able to recruit enough technically-proficient troops in order to operate its more sophisticated equipment, or even enough troops to maintain its current force design. South Africa is in the process of creating a database to determine the incidence of HIV in the armed forces, and the SANDF has recognised that it needs to change the sexual behaviour of its soldiers, and has initiated an education campaign against HIV in the military.[17]

Similar concerns are emerging among armed forces in Asia. The Vietnamese government considers AIDS as 'a natural calamity and enemy-inflicted destruction'.[18] John Chittick argues that, in Vietnam, 'it is feared that nations impacted greatly by HIV/AIDS will be seen as "weak" by neighboring countries and thus may be targeted as victims of military aggression'.[19] In Thailand, the military has designated HIV/AIDS a threat to national security.[20] According to Major-General Saksin Tipyakaysorn, chief of the Reserve Affairs Department, around 10% of conscripts in 1999, most of them from the northern and central plains, were found to be infected with HIV.[21] The military considers soldiers living with HIV or who are addicted to drugs a financial burden because the armed forces are responsible for their hospital treatment, and soldiers with HIV can be discharged from service.[22] In Cambodia, HIV/AIDS is 'cutting a swath through poorly educated military and police forces'.[23] Reports from Phnom Penh indicate that between 12% and 17% of armed forces personnel – national police and military – have HIV or AIDS, making them the second largest at-risk group after sex workers.[24] Dr Om Khantey, head of intensive care at the Preah Ket Mealea military hospital in Phnom Penh, has argued that HIV/AIDS 'is like the enemy of the people. There's no Khmer Rouge, now we have HIV'.[25] General Veng Bun Lay, chief of health for the Defence Ministry, insists that 'HIV/AIDS is now the military's only enemy, and this enemy is very difficult to fight'; HIV/AIDS 'could devastate our plans for reform and reduce our capability. We are very worried about this'.[26] Even China has begun testing military recruits for HIV.[27] The question that remains, however, is how serious this impact is likely to be strategically.

The strategic impact of high prevalence rates

Despite frequent claims to the contrary, there is no evidence that the impact of HIV/AIDS on armed forces is having strategic implications in the sense of inspiring or foreclosing the outbreak of armed conflicts. No armed conflicts have been initiated primarily because HIV/AIDS undermined a country's armed forces. This suggests that the strategic ramifications of the impact of HIV/AIDS on armed forces may be more complex than is commonly assumed, and its long-term effects dependent on a number of wider variables.

Identifying the key variables

At least two such variables can be identified. The first is the strategic environment of the states in question. A decrease in military capabilities will only become strategically significant if the environment is hostile, and there is a realistic chance that the armed forces will need to be fully used. In regions of relative stability or wealth, or where there is a culture of resolving conflicts through peaceful means, any impact on military capabilities is likely to be less relevant, perhaps even negligible, from a strategic perspective. Botswana, for example, has one of the highest HIV prevalence rates in the world, and yet has not seen significant armed conflict since the AIDS pandemic began to emerge. Thus, the strategic implications of HIV/AIDS in the country's armed forces are likely to be smaller than for a country in a more hostile environment. Similarly, the effect of HIV/AIDS is likely to be small if only a partial deployment of the armed forces is required. HIV/AIDS could only lead to novel armed conflicts by virtue of its impact on the armed forces if there were a reasonable chance of sustained armed conflict between two or more countries, and the impact on these two countries was significantly asymmetric. In many countries experiencing high prevalence rates, this is not the case. Nor does this type of conflict currently predominate in those areas worst affected by HIV/AIDS, where the larger challenge is typically internal and local.

The potential strategic implications of HIV/AIDS will also depend on the severity of its impact on armed forces in the long term. Some analysts have predicted that this impact will prove utterly overwhelming; one scholar, for example, argues that the disease will 'hollow out military capabilities' and weaken armed forces 'to the point of failure and collapse'.[28] Yet there is currently no sound evidence to corroborate such stark predictions. Based on the public information available, it is only possible to indicate with some confidence that HIV/AIDS poses novel challenges for the armed forces; it is not yet possible to tell precisely how serious this impact will become in future in terms of actual combat readiness. Such drastic assessments, in other words, are not only premature, but they also fail to appreciate the great diversity of the various armed forces in question, and the complex factors that will affect combat readiness. At least six factors will determine how severe the impact of HIV/AIDS on armed forces will become in the future: the level of HIV prevalence; the number of people who actually have AIDS; the type of armed forces involved;

levels of specialisation and technical proficiency; the size of the armed forces relative to the surrounding civilian population; and the level of leadership and resources available to address the problem.

In any given military, the degree of impact of HIV/AIDS will depend on the prevalence rates of HIV, as well as the absolute numbers involved. Given the high prevalence rates in Africa, these armed forces will need to be monitored particularly closely in the years ahead. Table 5 presents estimates of the number of affected people in selected African militaries, based on the percentage figures cited by the NIC.

Table 5: HIV Prevalence in Selected African Militaries

Country	Percentage	Total Active Armed Forces	Estimated with HIV/AIDS
Angola	40–60	130,500	52,000–78,000
Congo (Brazzaville)	10–25	10,000	1,000–2,500
Cote d'Ivoire	10–20	13,900	1,400–2,800
DRC	40–60	81,400	33,000–49,000
Eritrea	10	171,900	17,000
Nigeria	10–20	78,500	8,000–16,000
Tanzania	15–30	27,000	4,000–8,000

Source (total armed forces): *The Military Balance 2001–2002* (Oxford: Oxford University Press for the IISS, October 2001)

These figures indicate that, in countries where between 40% and 60% of the armed forces are thought to be HIV-positive, soldiers are expected to serve for a decade or more, and most of those who are HIV-positive develop AIDS within a decade, around half of the armed forces will have to be replaced over the next ten years if current staffing levels are to be maintained. In these circumstances, the impact on the armed forces will be severe. Even though militaries are used to making replacements on a continual basis, HIV/AIDS will significantly add to the number of replacements that would routinely have to be made for other reasons. At the same time, however, few militaries have such high prevalence rates; even for those with these high rates, not all of the soldiers who will eventually die of AIDS-related illnesses will have to be replaced at once. Where the prevalence rate is around 10%, the impact is likely to be less drastic, especially if taken into account in long-term planning.

It is also important to bear in mind that the number of soldiers in the front line is usually much smaller than the total number of active-service personnel; it is conceivable that the main impact of HIV/AIDS will be felt behind the front lines, in the support operations of the armed forces, to which sick soldiers might have been redeployed. This would still be a serious issue given that support operations are often crucial to the survival and combat effectiveness of front-line troops, but it is qualitatively different from claiming that the armed forces will collapse due to HIV/AIDS, or that their combat effectiveness will be severely diminished. In many African countries, due to other constraints, only a small proportion of the armed forces are deployable at short notice anyway.

The impact of HIV/AIDS on the capabilities of any given military will depend not only on the number of people in the armed forces who are HIV-positive, but also, and more importantly, on the number of people who actually have AIDS, and the number likely to develop AIDS in the near future. This figure can be significantly lower than HIV prevalence because of the lengthy illness cycle. In many cases, a soldier who is HIV-positive can still carry out most of his duties quite well, and HIV status alone is thus not an immediate, but a longer-term, concern for military capabilities. To predict the number of people who will develop AIDS, it would be necessary to know not only how many are HIV-positive, but also when they became HIV-positive, the average incubation periods for soldiers, and the average length of service. This kind of data is currently not publicly available, even if it exists. Depending on the time of infection and the average length of service of the militaries in question, a significant proportion of members could leave the armed forces before they develop AIDS.

The extent of the impact of HIV/AIDS on the military may also depend on the type of armed forces involved. There are interesting questions that still need to be researched around whether conscript and professional armies are affected in the same way and in equal measure by high levels of HIV/AIDS. Although both types of military structure are likely to encounter problems with long-serving staff due to reductions in average life expectancy, especially at the higher levels of the chain of command, they are likely to face different difficulties regarding short-term recruitment. Table 6 shows the estimated number of young men aged between 18 and 32 in selected countries affected by HIV/AIDS.

Table 6: Estimated numbers of young men in selected countries affected by HIV/AIDS

Country	Men Aged 18–22	Men Aged 23–32
Angola	583,000	888,000
Congo (Brazzaville)	148,000	234,000
Côte d'Ivoire	842,000	1,212,000
Democratic Republic of Congo	2,510,000	3,620,000
Eritrea	210,000	319,000
Nigeria	6,693,000	10,056,000
Tanzania	1,600,000	2,380,000

Source: The Military Balance 2001–2002

Armed forces with voluntary service will have to compete with other sectors of society for surviving young men. However, in the case of conscription forces, which often have terms of service ranging between six and 24 months, many conscripts will have left the armed forces before they develop full-blown AIDS, with the result that the implications for the armed forces would be less drastic.

A fourth important variable is the level of specialisation and technological proficiency. It is likely that those armed forces with more sophisticated communications and weapons systems will face graver problems in this regard than more basic forces, given the longer time that is needed to train soldiers, and the considerable expense involved. Indeed, there might even be important variations regarding the different branches of the armed forces. It is conceivable, for example, that given identical prevalence rates a state's air force will be affected relatively more severely than its army because training requirements are higher for pilots, and personnel cannot be replaced as easily or as quickly as basic foot soldiers. At the same time, many of the armed forces currently experiencing high prevalence rates are not amongst the technologically most sophisticated, and are not overly reliant on highly specialised training.

The impact of HIV/AIDS on the armed forces will also depend on the size of the military relative to the population as a whole. All things being equal, a small army in a populous country will have a large pool from which to draw new recruits, while a large army in a sparsely populated country is probably going to have much greater difficulties accommodating losses due to HIV/AIDS. Many African militaries are relatively small, with an estimated average in 1999 of 2.6 soldiers per 1,000 people. In southern Africa, the figure is even lower, at 1.7.[29] At the same time, small armies can be very capital intensive, thus making the loss of personnel due to HIV/AIDS more costly. Moreover, if a small army is responsible for covering a large territory, even minor factors affecting operational efficiency could have more significant strategic ramifications for a military's ability to effectively control this territory.

Finally, the impact of HIV/AIDS on the armed forces in the long term will also depend on the leadership available and the financial and medical resources that can be expended on addressing HIV/AIDS. Preliminary evidence indicates that, in those armed forces where the issue is addressed openly and responsibly, levels of new HIV infection can be reduced, and some of the tensions that HIV/AIDS can give rise to can be mitigated.

These are some of the important variables that will need to be considered when carrying out strategic assessments for individual armed forces. The complexity of these variables shows that one must be careful about making generalisations regarding the impact of HIV/AIDS on armed forces. While HIV/AIDS is likely to confront armed forces with real and important new challenges in years to come, especially in those militaries with very high prevalence rates, the magnitude and impact of HIV/AIDS will vary considerably from military to military, depending on the particular mix of the factors outlined above.

Exploring possible scenarios

Even if the two main variables identified above intersect – if losses due to HIV/AIDS impinge on the armed forces' combat readiness, and if the country involved is in a pervasively hostile strategic environment – the relationship between HIV/AIDS and the possible outbreak of armed conflict would still be complex, and certainly much less straightforward than is often suggested. On balance, it is unlikely that HIV/AIDS will generate new armed conflicts solely on the basis of its impact on armed forces.

Hypothetically, there are at least two ways in which HIV/AIDS could create novel incentives for conflict, neither of which is very likely. First, a decrease in military capacity could theoretically increase a state's vulnerability to external attack, or its vulnerability to internal rebel groups. A perceived weakness in a military force due to high levels of AIDS might conceivably lead another country to launch an offensive from which it might otherwise have been deterred. This risk is exacerbated if the impact of HIV/AIDS on two neighbouring countries is asymmetrical over time. To the extent that there are regional variations in the impact of HIV/AIDS on armed forces, strategic balances could thus become unhinged, increasing the likelihood of armed conflict. The defence analyst Paul Beaver, for example, has argued that the AIDS pandemic might contribute to the outbreak of war by encouraging one state to attack another in the belief that high HIV prevalence would render that state's armed forces less effective.[30] In this instance, the perception that a state is being hit particularly severely by HIV/AIDS may be as important as the pandemic's actual impact.

These kinds of incentives would not necessarily be confined to Africa. According to John Chittick, in Vietnam AIDS is a cause of concern in the light of the history of conflict between Vietnam and China, over border issues and the disputed ownership of the Spratly Islands in the South China Sea. Vietnam thus continues to link its security with a strong and regular supply of young recruits.[31] In October 1990, the threat that AIDS posed to this supply was deemed great enough to prompt the establishment of a National AIDS Committee. According to Chittick, 'the defense capabilities of a smaller populated nation might be more adversely affected than that of a country with a population 15 times greater' due to AIDS.[32] In other words, HIV/AIDS could become strategically relevant by having an asymmetric impact on two countries with antagonistic relations, and could thus shift the balance of power in favour of one party, thereby increasing the incentive for either an offensive war, or a defensive war to prevent a future attack when the military will be weakened even further.

Important factors raise considerable doubts as to whether this incentive could ever suffice to contribute to the outbreak of conflict. Firstly, there is the regional nature of the spread of HIV/AIDS, and the important role of proximity in armed conflicts. It is likely that, if one country is affected by prevalence rates high enough to have an impact on its military capabilities, its neighbours will have much the same problems. In Sub-Saharan Africa in particular, many countries are facing similarly high prevalence rates, as are contending groups within countries. Thus, in Sierra Leone Major Olu Cleeve, the chief medical officer at Freetown's military hospital, believes that the prevalence rate among rebels is probably roughly the same as that in the SLA (though obtaining information on HIV prevalence amongst rebel groups is often even more difficult than getting such information about regular forces).[33] In this case, the difference between parties would not be expected to be that great, unless one party to a potential dispute has been able to reduce prevalence significantly, or because a country has a substantially smaller population from which to staff its armed forces.

Even if a considerable discrepancy in the balance of power does emerge over time, it is hard to identify any historical precedents where the prevalence of disease alone caused the outbreak of conflict. Induction, of course, is not foolproof, but it does raise questions about whether the prevalence of HIV/AIDS alone is sufficient for the outbreak of armed conflict, and it does cast doubt on the scenario of a state initiating armed conflict on only these grounds. Even in the case of Vietnam mentioned by Chittick, it seems that the force discrepancy with China is significant enough in and of itself to make HIV/AIDS a much less significant factor compared to other variables in determining and constraining any confrontation between the two countries. The deployment of armed force always occurs in a larger political context, and discrepancies in force strength alone are rarely the only reason for the outbreak of conflict. In Africa, HIV/AIDS is similarly not the only factor determining force strength. Many other issues, such as declining military budgets, the reduction in external military aid following the end of the Cold War and international pressures to demobilise are also important. Nor, for that matter, is there a direct relationship between manpower and combat effectiveness. In recent African conflicts, many soldiers have switched sides, and mobilisation rates have been very low even before HIV/AIDS is taken into account. Only a relatively small proportion of the armed forces will actually participate in combat. Not only is it unclear whether combat capabilities will actually be significantly diminished by HIV/AIDS, but other political and strategic factors are likely to be much more important and decisive than HIV prevalence. HIV/AIDS is thus unlikely to generate new wars along these lines.

The second way in which HIV/AIDS could conceivably create novel incentives for the deployment of armed force is that armed forces, or parts thereof, might use conflict in order to capture or loot resources to pay for their own medications. Africa has witnessed many conflicts aimed at capturing resources such as diamonds, gold and timber. Often the loyalty of troops may have more to do with such opportunities for looting than with any ethnic or ideological motive.[34] Given the availability of expensive medicines, AIDS creates powerful new incentives to obtain resources, if only to prolong one's life. Soldiers who are knowledgeable about their HIV status are understandably concerned about the illness. In fact, the desperation of many is clearly evident. Nigerian soldiers returning from missions in Liberia and Sierra Leone with HIV are reported to have been seeking out the 'miraculous' healing powers of Prophet Joshua in the Synagogue Church of All Nations in Lagos.[35] In the DRC, there have been allegations of looting, possibly in part to finance expensive AIDS therapies.

Yet here too there is considerable room for scepticism as to whether this incentive will actually prove powerful enough to animate new conflicts. First, there are no confirmed examples of this occurring, and this scenario is based on logical deduction and rumour. Second, even if the rumours from the DRC are corroborated, this would not be a case of a conflict started for this reason, only of a conflict that was possibly not resolved as quickly as it might otherwise have been. Finally, HIV/AIDS would only be one factor amongst many others that would make such looting worthwhile, and it is not even evident that it would be the most important.

While it is certainly true that the impact of HIV/AIDS could, in some cases, create important new incentives for the deployment of armed force, it does not follow from the emergence of these incentives alone that such armed conflicts will actually occur. These novel incentives, after all, will always have to be judged in the larger context of competing constraints and incentives for not deploying armed force. The argument that HIV/AIDS will cause novel conflicts because of its impact on armed forces is tenuous at best, relying mostly on logical deduction rather than on empirically observed, or historically corroborated, phenomena.

In fact, high prevalence rates amongst armed forces could conceivably have benign strategic effects. This possibility is usually ignored in discussions of the strategic implications of HIV/AIDS. A reduction in operational efficiency could, for example, hamper expansive and offensive military plans in bellicose countries. In effect, any AIDS-related reduction in military capabilities would cut both ways: although it might increase one state's vulnerability to outside attack, it could also inhibit another's expansionist plans. Second, weakened armed forces may not be such a negative development in countries where the military is corrupt, repressive or opposed to democratisation processes. In such countries, not everyone would necessarily lament a weakened capability amongst the armed forces, although much would of course depend on how the military responds to its weakening position. Neither of these possibilities would do anything to diminish the humanitarian implications of high prevalence rates, but they do show that the question of whether these prevalence rates will have strategic implications by virtue of their impact on armed forces is much more complex than commonly assumed.

The scenarios that could arise from the impact of HIV/AIDS on armed forces are clearly multiple and complex, and this should caution analysts against drawing a clear relationship between the impact of HIV/AIDS on the military and the outbreak of new armed conflicts. HIV/AIDS might create important new incentives for the deployment of armed force, and these must be recognised; but it also creates new disincentives that equally should not be overlooked. Moreover, the new incentives that HIV/AIDS creates would only become significant in a hostile strategic environment and, even then, many other political, legal, economic and social factors are likely to be more decisive than HIV prevalence in encouraging or constraining the deployment of armed force.

Conclusion

The fact that HIV/AIDS is unlikely to generate new armed conflicts does not mean that it does not have considerable strategic import. The emerging evidence from African militaries in particular suggests clearly that the AIDS pandemic has an important strategic dimension in that it poses difficult new challenges for armed forces. These challenges are already significant in Africa; they are also faced, to a lesser extent, by armed forces around the world. This impact will become amplified in the years to come, and as mortality rates increase. Armed forces do not stand outside the AIDS pandemic, but, like most sectors of societies, are profoundly affected by it. The higher the military prevalence rate, and the longer it has been consistently high, the more severe the problems faced by armed forces will become. In the worst-affected countries, the armed forces are likely to confront an increasingly unhealthy conscription pool, to lose technically-qualified and specialised personnel prematurely, to experience losses at all levels within the command structure, and to incur additional costs in treating soldiers living with AIDS. Even when such personnel can be replaced, this can only be done at additional cost. These aspects of HIV/AIDS are far from trivial, and are already affecting the operational efficiency of many armed forces. In this way, HIV/AIDS clearly has a strategic dimension, and this will have to be taken seriously in the years ahead.

This does not, however, imply that armed forces will become completely hollowed out or will collapse under the additional challenges posed by HIV/AIDS. It is too early to determine with confidence exactly how seriously HIV/AIDS will undermine the capabilities of armed forces in the years to come; information is scarce, there is great fluctuation in prevalence rates between different armed forces, and the strategic environments and force designs of individual states vary significantly. Consequently, there is a clear need for more extensive and country-specific research into the impact of HIV/AIDS on the military capabilities of specific armed forces, focusing more closely on this set of variables. To date, the only systematic and public research being done on African militaries is on the South African National Defence Force, and the findings are not readily applicable to other armed forces in Africa or elsewhere.

Chapter 3

HIV/AIDS and peacekeeping operations

Many armed forces with high HIV prevalence rates also regularly contribute to international peacekeeping operations aimed at mitigating and containing the outbreak of armed conflicts. In this way HIV/AIDS has additional strategic ramifications in the international realm. A decrease in overall military capability could not only affect a country's ability to defend itself against outside threats, but could also impede its ability to project power abroad and to contribute to non-essential missions such as peacekeeping. HIV/AIDS poses additional logistical and political problems for these operations, as it becomes increasingly well known that peacekeepers are at special risk of contracting and spreading HIV.[1]

HIV/AIDS has begun to affect international peacekeeping operations in five important ways. First, peacekeepers have acted as vectors of HIV, spreading the virus among populations in areas of deployment. Second, the risk of forces contracting HIV while on deployment may reduce a contributing state's willingness to participate in peacekeeping operations. Third, HIV/AIDS prevalence among contributing forces may make it more difficult to staff operations. Fourth, states may become less willing to host peacekeeping missions. Finally, the constrained capacity of states to contribute to peacekeeping missions may create additional resource difficulties as the earning potential of such operations is reduced.

Peacekeepers as vectors of HIV

HIV/AIDS poses new challenges for regional and international peacekeeping operations as countries recognise that such operations may contribute to the spread of HIV/AIDS. 'Here,' Richard Holbrooke has argued, 'we get into one of the ugliest secret truths ... about AIDS: it is spread by UN peacekeepers.'[2] In Holbrooke's view, this creates 'almost the greatest irony of all: in the cause of peacekeeping to spread a disease which is killing 10 times as many people as war'.[3] In Sierra Leone, the presence of peacekeepers from armies where prevalence rates are high, such as Zambia, Kenya and Nigeria, appears to have increased the number of infections.[4] According to one report, '32 percent of peacekeepers [in Sierra Leone] originate from countries with HIV prevalence rates greater than 5 percent'.[5] Sixty women have tested HIV-positive in Kossoh Town, on the outskirts of Freetown, where the ECOMOG headquarters were based. The prevalence of HIV in the area is widely thought to be linked to the large number of sex workers that the ECOMOG presence attracted.[6]

Similar problems have emerged in Cambodia, where HIV prevalence rates appear to have increased dramatically following the arrival of the UN Transitional Authority in Cambodia (UNTAC) in 1992–93.[7] By the end of 1999, an estimated 220,000 people were living with HIV, and the prevalence rate was 4.04%. Although there is insufficient data to prove the case, officials in Phnom Penh place considerable blame for the spread of the epidemic on UNTAC.[8] Holbrooke also points out that East Timor 'never had a reported case of AIDS until the UN got there. I'm not saying there weren't any cases because it's a remote area but we now have 20 reported cases. In a population of 800,000, that's significant.'[9] In addition to voluntary and commercial sexual encounters, there have been several reported incidents of sexual abuse committed by peacekeepers. Between the 1992 peace accord and the 1994 elections in Mozambique, for example, there were numerous reports of sexual abuse of women and children by UN peacekeepers.[10]

Peacekeepers are rarely the only source for spreading infection, and it is actually very difficult to quantify this problem because many of the epidemiological preconditions cannot be properly met in areas where peacekeepers are deployed; the UN Department of Peacekeeping Operations (DPKO) does not know the number of HIV-positive soldiers deployed in peacekeeping missions. There have, however, been six confirmed HIV-positive peacekeepers deployed in East Timor, and another six in Kosovo, though it is unclear whether they were so prior to deployment.[11]

Willingness to contribute to international peacekeeping operations

Peacekeepers are also at risk of acquiring HIV/AIDS from civilians in the countries to which they are deployed. Many of the factors that render national military populations a high-risk group in terms of HIV/AIDS apply equally to international peacekeepers. Peacekeepers may be posted away from home for long periods of time. Some Nigerian peacekeepers, for example, were reportedly on field duty, without rotation, for up to three years as part of *Operation Sandstorm* in Sierra Leone. In this instance, the HIV incidence rate was also correlated with the length of duty, increasing from 7% after one year, to 10% after two years and to 15% after three.[12] Peacekeeping missions also tend to attract large numbers of sex workers, thus linking two high-risk groups.[13] In Cambodia, UNTAC brought more than 20,000 foreign military and civilian personnel into Cambodia. Large amounts of money poured into a country ravaged by poverty. Sex workers, some from as far afield as Eastern Europe, apparently doubled the number of clients per night, from five to ten.

HIV/AIDS may make peacekeeping missions increasingly unpopular among contributing countries.[14] Countries may become reluctant to contribute to operations if they believe that large numbers of personnel will return HIV-positive. Of the 10,000 troops that Nigeria sent to Sierra Leone in 1997, 11% of those who returned tested HIV-positive.[15] The Nigerian government admitted in December 1999 that there was an extremely high prevalence rate amongst its troops participating in ECOMOG operations in neighbouring West African states.[16] Although specific figures were not given, Vice-President Abubakar Atiku described the situation as 'grave'. Since the 1980s, more peacekeepers have succumbed to AIDS-related illnesses than to battle injuries.[17] Peacekeepers deployed from Western countries have also been affected; Finnish soldiers on a tour of duty in Namibia in the early 1990s, for instance, were infected with HIV.[18] Troops from Europe, Asia and North America became infected with HIV during the UN mission in Cambodia from 1993; 45 Indian soldiers tested positive for HIV on their return, as did two from Bangladesh, one from Mozambique and ten from Uruguay.[19] Western troops serving in Bosnia have reportedly contracted the illness.[20] Given that peacekeepers are often stationed far from their home countries, they may bring home new and different strands of HIV. Tests on returning UNTAC soldiers from the US and Uruguay, for example, revealed infection with the HIV subtype E, which had previously only been found in Southeast Asia and Central Africa.[21]

Ability to staff peacekeeping operations

Individual peacekeeping operations may also come under increasing staffing pressure as HIV prevalence rates rise in national armies. Peacekeeping operations can be notoriously difficult to staff. Depending on the conflicts involved, it is not always easy for the UN to find sufficient peacekeepers to meet its operational demands, and the DPKO cannot always be as choosy as it might like. This problem is further exacerbated by HIV/AIDS, which could lead to a decrease in the number of personnel that states can contribute to such operations.[22] Greg Mills, director of the South African Institute of International Affairs, has studied this problem in relation to the Southern Africa Development Community (SADC). During the SADC Blue Crane peacekeeping exercise in South Africa in April 1999, nearly 50% of the 4,500 participating troops were HIV-positive; 30% of the South African contingent was not medically fit for deployment.[23] Mills argues that:

> *the high rate of infection in SADC armies also calls into question the nature and size of their potential contribution to a Congo mission. In more general terms, it presents problems for and questions the appropriateness of the current Western strategy to devolve the responsibility for peacekeeping missions down to the sub-regional level in Africa. Preliminary studies of an SANDF peacekeeping operation in the Democratic Republic of Congo (DRC) suggest that the military contingent will be far more at risk from disease than bullets.*[24]

According to one analyst at the Institute for Security Studies, several countries including South Africa might be unable to participate in peacekeeping operations in the future, at least not to the extent that they have in the past.[25] The SANDF has grave concerns about its ability to find enough volunteers for its international peacekeeping commitments, particularly given UN recommendations to test all peacekeepers prior to deployment.[26] HIV-positive soldiers may not be suitable for peacekeeping operations, especially when they are being deployed to areas where adequate medical facilities are not available.

According to Deputy Defence Minister Nozizwe Madlala-Routledge, HIV/AIDS poses a threat not only to peace and security in South Africa, but for Africa at large: 'South Africa must be able to fulfil its obligations toward its people as well as the international community', and this 'is only possible through healthy and motivated soldiers'.[27]

Willingness to host peacekeeping operations

HIV/AIDS may limit not only the cooperation of those countries contributing to peacekeeping operations, but also of those hosting such missions. In March 2001, for example, the Eritrean government requested that peacekeepers deployed to the country should be screened for HIV, and demanded a guarantee from the UN that no HIV-positive soldiers would be deployed.[28] This political problem was exacerbated by subsequent allegations that one peacekeeper sexually abused an under-age girl.[29] In Sierra Leone, United Nations HIV/AIDS coordinator Hirut Befecadu has insisted that 'the population should be protected from the soldiers as well, because most of the troops come from places where AIDS is a problem'.[30] During the Balkans conflicts, officials in Zagreb sought to ensure that no African peacekeepers served in Croatia in light of the risk of HIV transmission.[31] One report in 2001 has suggested that the 'concern that foreign peacekeeping troops may carry the virus may prompt populations to reject cooperation with such forces, contributing to the continuation of conflict'.[32] Although this is going too far, it may be the case that peacekeeping contingents may no longer be seen as neutral and benign, but rather as bringing with them novel political complications.

The UN Security Council has begun to take this issue seriously enough to address it formally by passing Resolution 1308, which urges, but does not compel, member states to screen their soldiers. It also calls upon the Secretary-General to provide pre-deployment orientation for peacekeepers on preventing the spread of HIV. In 2001, soldiers from the UN mission in Eritrea and Ethiopia completed the first two-week AIDS-prevention course to be offered to peacekeepers.[33] The UN has bought over 1.5m condoms for its peacekeepers in Sierra Leone and East Timor (rationed to one condom per peacekeeper per day), and has distributed 15,000 AIDS-awareness cards.[34] However, using only disease-free peacekeepers is in practice difficult given human-rights considerations, and the UN's reliance on certain armed forces to meet operational requirements.

The resource dimension

For many countries, contributing to peacekeeping operations is seen as a way of obtaining additional funds for armed forces and defence ministries.[35] Peacekeeping operations are one way for poor countries to obtain vital foreign currency. As of September 2001, countries contributing peacekeepers to UN missions around the world were being reimbursed at around $1,000 per peacekeeper per month; this figure is likely to have increased since.[36] Yet many of these militaries also have high HIV prevalence rates.[37] If for this reason they are no longer able to participate in peacekeeping operations, they will lose important resources.

Conclusion

Although there is currently no way of quantifying the phenomenon, and ascertaining to what extent peacekeepers spread the virus, HIV/AIDS clearly presents a novel set of operational and political challenges for the maintenance of international peace and security. In this sense, HIV/AIDS has another important and emerging strategic dimension. This emerging impact on international peacekeeping operations means that high HIV prevalence rates in African and Asian armed forces are not only of concern to the individual countries affected. Given that many of these armed forces also contribute to international peacekeeping operations, Western countries are also affected by these trends. If countries such as Nigeria and South Africa experience difficulties in the long term, this will have important implications for the stability of the region more generally, given the contribution these countries could make to peacekeeping in Africa.

It seems unlikely that high HIV prevalence in a particular country will single-handedly influence decisions to deploy peacekeeping forces; the British, for instance, sent forces to Sierra Leone to broker a peace, even if attempts to rebuild the country's armed forces were not helped by the high HIV prevalence in its army. Nevertheless, the British Ministry of Defence predicts that HIV/AIDS will become an 'increasingly important consideration' for the soldiers that it deploys abroad.[38] It will thus be necessary to continue tracing this strategic dimension of HIV/AIDS closely in the years to come.

Chapter 4

HIV/AIDS and political stability

In countries where HIV prevalence rates are highest, the strategic dimension of the AIDS pandemic is not confined exclusively to its narrower impact on the armed forces. In these countries, many of which are in Africa, HIV/AIDS could also have broader, long-term implications for political stability. As early as 1990, the CIA added AIDS incidence to the list of variables that should be considered when analysing which states were likely to become unstable or collapse in future.[1] In December 2001, a report by UNAIDS noted that, in Sub-Saharan Africa, the 'risks of social unrest and even socio-political instability should not be under-estimated'.[2]

The long-term social consequences of HIV/AIDS would certainly add to the gravity of the current health problem. There are historical precedents; Zinsser, writing in the 1930s, noted that whenever illnesses have reached great magnitudes, 'their secondary consequences have been much more far-reaching and disorganizing than anything that could have resulted from the mere numerical reduction of the population'.[3] Widespread illnesses have not only produced panic, but additionally bred 'social and moral disorganization; farms were abandoned, and there was shortage of food; famine led to displacement of populations, to revolution, to civil war'.[4] As recently as September 1994, when pneumonic plague broke out in the Indian town of Surat, around a quarter of the population fled in panic within four days.

HIV/AIDS is unlikely to have such immediate effects in light of its long cycle, but if instability were to be replicated cumulatively in the long run, this would be strategically significant not only for regions directly affected, but also for states with interests in these regions and for those charged with maintaining international peace and security. Such political instability could affect regimes that are friendly to the West, or ones that are undergoing democratisation, and instability in any one state could have knock-on effects on neighbouring states, potentially requiring outside intervention. Yet, as with the case of the armed forces, the processes through which HIV/AIDS might lead to political instability and state collapse are far more complex than is usually acknowledged, and there is a similar lack of detailed research. As one scholar has correctly noted, 'research – on a topic which is crucial for the survival of democratic governance in some countries – has simply not yet begun'.[5] The key question will be one of degree. Is HIV/AIDS likely just to generate novel challenges that increase the difficulty of maintaining political stability in the worst-affected countries? Or is it also likely, in some cases, to precipitate in state collapse?

When states become unstable or fail, it is usually because the central monopoly on the use of armed force is disputed, and because the government's popular legitimacy has been severely eroded. Such processes of state collapse do not necessarily occur instantaneously, but can, as William Zartmann has argued, be likened to 'a long-term degenerative disease'.[6] State collapse is normally a multi-faceted phenomenon involving at least three interrelated processes. First, the economy is transformed or destroyed and there is an increase in crime. Second, political institutions dissolve at both the local and national level. Third, social institutions such as the family, the education system or health care are damaged.[7] High rates of HIV and AIDS contribute to all three of these processes. As such, the growing AIDS pandemic also emerges as a matter of considerable concern in the long term, especially for the political stability of states that are already weak or facing complex emergencies.

Competition for resources

HIV/AIDS contributes to the first trajectory involved in state collapse in that care for sufferers adds to the resource burden countries face, and intensifies competition over scarce resources. The findings of the previous two chapters provide a useful starting point in this regard. The armed forces are likely to try to secure a greater share of public expenditure in order to offset these emerging resource demands. In southern Africa, Namibian Deputy Minister of Defence Victor Simunja has expressed serious concern about the resource burden that HIV/AIDS poses for the Namibian military, arguing that the cost of caring for affected military personnel 'is likely to increase significantly in the coming years'.[8]

The civilian sector will similarly face an increased resource demand. According to one study, in 1997 more than 2% of gross domestic product (GDP) was used for public-health spending towards HIV/AIDS in seven of 16 African countries sampled. These are countries where traditionally total health spending accounts for around 3% to 5% of GDP.[9] In the mid-1990s, it was estimated that 66% of Rwanda's health budget and over a quarter of Zimbabwe's went on treatment for people with HIV.[10] In Malawi, the public health system is already inundated by the pandemic, with up to 70% of hospital beds occupied by patients suffering from AIDS-related illnesses. In light of the scarcity of resources, funds are being diverted from treating other illnesses. In Kenya, for example, mortality among patients with other illnesses is growing because they are being admitted at later stages of their illness.[11] Zimbabwe has introduced a 3% tax on personal and corporate income in order to fund a trust for people living with HIV.[12]

According to a report published by the NIC in the US, the worst-affected countries will also suffer from a reduction in economic growth of up to 1% of GDP per annum due to AIDS, and the disease will consume more than half of the health budgets of these countries.[13] The Secretary-General of the UN reports that, in the next 20 years, the worst-affected countries could well lose up to a quarter of their projected economic growth.[14] In a Sub-Saharan African country with a prevalence rate of around 20%, annual GDP growth would be 2.6% lower.[15] A recent World Health Organisation (WHO) report conservatively estimates that the economic value of the lives lost due to AIDS in Sub-Saharan Africa is equivalent to 11% of the region's combined gross national product in 1999.[16] While these kinds of losses could be absorbed for a year or two, they pose larger problems when they become cumulative, occurring year after year as they are likely to do. HIV/AIDS affects the economically most productive demographic group and undermines belief in the long-term sustainability of the economy, and so could discourage private as well as foreign investment.

This increased burden could intensify the competition for public resources between the military and civilian sectors. In South Africa, for example, military expenditure decreased from 13.1% of government spending in 1989 to 6.8% in 1995. Yet many segments of the civilian population take issue with defence expenditure of even this size in light of the growing AIDS epidemic that the country is facing. In 1998, the cabinet's decision to authorise a costly weapon-procurement programme attracted severe and widespread public criticism.[17] In Cambodia, the decision not to use the 'peace dividend' to increase funding for social services similarly led to heated political debate. While there was a marginal increase in such funding in the 2000 budget, security and defence spending still amounted to around 59% of total expenditure, which represents only a modest cut compared to 1999. Opposition leader Sam Rainsy argued that this was tantamount to the government 'stealing 20 years from each person. The government is stealing the people's money and lives'.[18]

It will not be easy to alleviate these resource tensions given that the most productive sector of affected economies in Sub-Saharan Africa, namely the extractive industry, is itself important in the spread of HIV/AIDS. Miners in particular constitute a high-risk group. Often, mining sites are far removed from urban areas and tend to attract sex workers with very high prevalence rates. One survey conducted in a gold-mining area near Johannesburg found that, of 88,000 miners, 20% were HIV-positive, as were 75% of the 400–500 sex workers.[19] As a result, 'a severe AIDS epidemic seriously threatens domestically retained and reinvested mining revenues at all levels of present and future production'.[20] Truck drivers form another high-risk group; the transportation of goods over long distances is crucial to a functioning and expanding economy, but it also facilitates the spread of the illness. Drivers can be on the road for weeks at a time, often seeking casual sexual encounters at rest stops along the highways.

HIV/AIDS is also closely linked to rapid economic modernisation and to natural resource extraction, which will make the economic losses generated by high prevalence rates much more difficult to offset in the long run. The resource burden is going to prove particularly intractable for the worst-affected countries without some form of support from the international community. Given that HIV/AIDS affects not only the poor, but also the skilled workers who are in short supply in many countries, HIV/AIDS is unlikely to produce the same economic benefits for the survivors that the bubonic plague is thought by some historians to have provided, through raising wages and depressing land prices. This is particularly true for economies integrated into the global economy, where investment capital might easily move to regions with lower morbidity and mortality rates.[21]

Political tensions

HIV/AIDS may also contribute to state collapse by generating additional challenges to the political sphere in countries where prevalence rates are high.

AIDS and governance

First, HIV/AIDS could further undermine the capacity of states to govern effectively. Crucial resources are already being diverted from state services to treating people with HIV/AIDS. In Tanzania, for example, over half of the expenses designated for administrative costs for the Harbours Authority were reportedly diverted to addressing the costs of HIV/AIDS in 2000.[22] Basic services will become increasingly difficult to deliver as mortality rates increase. Namibia, for example, depends on purified water, yet the largest purification company, NamWater, is reported to have operational difficulties due to the impact of HIV/AIDS on its workforce.[23] A representative of the UK's development assistance organisation Crown Agents has observed that 'we have experienced reductions in staff resources in a counterpart government department in excess of 50 percent in less than 12 months in one central southern African country, and between 25 and 50 per cent in other countries'.[24] As a matter of urgency, it will be necessary to gather data on whether such figures are typical.

In many countries with high prevalence rates, the police are coming under increasing pressure. The police forces of the 14 SADC countries are trying to find ways to cope with the reduction in personnel, and are bracing themselves for much worse in the years to come.[25] In Kenya, AIDS caused 75% of deaths in the police force between 1998 and 2000, and the Zambian police force is reported to have felt a similarly severe impact from HIV/AIDS.[26] All things being equal, this means that in future it will become more difficult to fight crime and fewer arrests will probably be made. It will also become more difficult to handle internal rebellions or other domestic challenges to state authority.

In the years to come, HIV/AIDS could significantly complicate the governing process of the state by affecting its institutions at local and national levels. According to one study, a pregnant Rwandan in 1987 had 'a 9 percent chance of being HIV positive if her husband was a farmer, a 22 percent chance if he was in the army, and a 38 percent chance if he worked for the government'.[27] AIDS does not affect only the lower levels of a state's bureaucracy; in several countries, it is thought to have first appeared amongst the wealthier and more educated social groups. AIDS will thus also lead to the death of top-level political leaders, or will prevent such individuals from seeking office. In Zimbabwe, three government ministers have already died from AIDS-related illnesses, and six are reported to be HIV-positive.[28] To some extent, access to expensive medicines and treatment is easier for people at the higher end of the government hierarchy, but even the former Zambian President Kenneth Kaunda could not prevent his son's AIDS death.

These problems could be exacerbated if the tax base erodes. HIV/AIDS targets those income groups most likely to pay taxes, as well as the poor. People might begin to refuse to pay taxes in the light of their own declining social and economic situation, or if they begin to disengage with a government perceived not to be looking after even their most basic interests, namely physical survival.

Reconfiguring political power

HIV/AIDS could also influence long-term political events in regions where political stability currently rests on fragile alliances between different antagonistic political groups, or where power lies in the hands of a small elite. Tensions could emerge if one group felt itself to be disproportionately affected, and believed that other groups were deliberately not doing enough to address the issue. In Uganda in the mid-1990s, for example, the defence minister is alleged to have suggested that one of the most likely potential triggers for a coup was the perception among the military that the government was not doing enough to combat HIV/AIDS.[29]

Ruling groups have in the past been willing to manipulate crises such as famines to target and weaken others. In Sudan, for example, government forces have frequently attacked health centres and food distribution centres catering to opponents, and have attempted to deny their opponents access to food.[30] Similarly, the different impact of HIV/AIDS on different groups could in the long run become part of a political calculus, producing demographic shifts. This impact would not necessarily have to be drastic in order to be politically relevant. Even where individuals are not yet visibly ill, HIV/AIDS can be politicised, for instance during elections. In the run-up to general elections in Zambia in December 2001, the government considered a bill that would compel presidential candidates to undergo HIV tests. As Brigadier-General Godfrey Miyanda, the presidential candidate of the opposition Heritage party, noted at the time, 'as much as it is proper to ensure that all presidential candidates are in a healthy state, the timing of this bill is rather suspicious'.[31] In all likelihood, the intent of the bill was to marginalise candidates who were HIV-positive. Several politicians have associated HIV/AIDS with economic migrants as a way of increasing their political influence, or in order to find scapegoats for their country's high prevalence rates.

Access to medicines

HIV/AIDS could also generate political tensions over access to life-saving medicines. Diseases have ravaged many countries for decades without necessarily leading to political instability. Yet, unlike other diseases that are closely linked with poverty, HIV/AIDS additionally afflicts the educated and moderately wealthy middle classes. Given the availability of anti-retroviral treatments for HIV/AIDS, many elites with access to resources will be able to substantially relieve their predicament by purchasing medicines. Indeed, for those amongst the elites who are HIV-positive, their illness could form a strong incentive not to relinquish this power. The fate of the middle classes is less certain. If elites are not seen to be working in their interests and securing medication for them as well, or if the middle classes cannot afford medication, this could contribute to further polarisation between the classes. Randy Cheek argues that the 'uneven distribution of essential HIV treatment based on social, ethnic, or political criteria could well put unmanageable pressures on social and political structures, threatening the stability of regimes throughout Southern Africa'.[32] The provision of medicines might become a central factor driving people's political loyalties; one of the primary reasons for South African President Thabo Mbeki's decline in popularity has been his reluctance to fund treatments for HIV, and this is thought to be provoking friction within the governing coalition.[33] Where medicines are not provided by the government, people may become increasingly susceptible to populist politicians promising radical solutions, at the expense of democratically-elected leaders.

Distracting from the AIDS pandemic

HIV/AIDS could potentially foster political instability if political leaders seek to generate disorder to distract from the devastating social impact of HIV/AIDS. One interesting relationship in this regard is the effect of HIV/AIDS on food supplies. In Zimbabwe, for instance, one analyst has suggested that:

> *Mugabe obviously is stoking the coals of the long-simmering land redistribution issue to distract the voters from other sources of dissatisfaction with his government. Unemployment in the country has reached 50 percent; inflation has risen to 70 percent. Fuel supplies are perilously low, and AIDS has reached epidemic proportions.*[34]

President Mugabe might well be utilising political disorder to distract from the many social problems ravaging Zimbabwe, including HIV/AIDS. This would be part of a larger tendency, analysed by Patrick Chabal and Jean-Pascal Daloz, of leaders exploiting confusion, uncertainty and disorder in order to accommodate their interests.[35] Even though AIDS may not yet be perceived as the most significant of these problems, it feeds back indirectly into more immediate difficulties; declining agricultural productivity, for example, can be traced to the impact of HIV/AIDS on the most productive age groups.

HIV/AIDS could thus pose additional, novel and serious challenges to political stability along at least four different trajectories. Again, however, one must be cautious about asserting a categorical and direct causality in this regard. The political relationships involved are elaborate and contingent. They also differ significantly between states, and one must be cautious in generalising about the African continent as a whole. Moreover, if such effects were to materialise in any country in future, they are more likely to be largely indirect and cumulative, than direct. This does not make them any less real or important, however. Some analysts, for example, have already raised the question of whether the security and stability of Mozambique can be maintained in the long term given that half of today's 15-year-olds in Maputo will be dead by the time they are 45.[36] To date, these four trajectories have not been properly explored; as Alan Whiteside rightly points out, 'as a matter of urgency we need to look at the effect the epidemic is having on the state sector ... on the ability of the state to actually function. Unfortunately, nobody has done this'.[37]

Social cohesion and civil society

In addition to the serious challenges that HIV/AIDS presents for a country's resources and for its efficient governance, it also has an important impact on the social cohesion of populations. This could become strategically significant if it challenges a state's monopoly on the use of armed force.

HIV/AIDS undermines a wide array of social institutions, including the family, the education system and the health sector. Given that social relations ultimately revolve around human beings, virtually no aspect of social life remains untouched by the illness in countries where the epidemic is prevalent and widespread. HIV/AIDS is already having a negative effect on the provision of education in many African countries, reducing the supply of teachers and consequently also the overall quality of education that can be provided. It is estimated that, in some regions in southern Africa, around a fifth of secondary-school teachers are HIV-positive, and some schools are being forced to close. In 1999, it was estimated that 860,000 primary-school children in Sub-Saharan Africa had lost teachers to AIDS.[38] AIDS is also likely to constrain the amount of public resources available for the education sector, as well as keeping many children out of school because their labour is needed to support their household.[39]

One of the starkest effects of the illness is that it leads to a drastic decrease in average life expectancy. The NIC estimates that the reduction in life expectancy will range from around three years in Thailand and four years in Haiti, to eight and 13 years in Brazil and Honduras respectively, and 20 years in South Africa and Nigeria. The countries worst hit will be Botswana and Zimbabwe, where life expectancy will decrease by 30 years.[40] The UN Development Programme provides slightly different figures, highlighting again the difficulties in making such calculations with great precision.

Table 7: Calculated loss of life expectancy due to HIV/AIDS in selected countries, as estimated by UNDP, 1999

Country	2010–2015 Life Expectancy at Birth		
	Expected (with AIDS)	Hypothetical (without AIDS)	Years of Life Expectancy Lost
Namibia	41.5	67.7	26.3
Botswana	48.9	73.0	24.1
South Africa	47.2	67.4	20.1
Zimbabwe	50.4	69.8	19.4
Kenya	51.0	69.8	18.8
Mozambique	39.6	56.7	17.1
Zambia	51.5	63.7	12.3
Cameroon	55.3	66.2	10.9
Tanzania	52.4	63.2	10.8
Malawi	48.1	57.3	9.2
Lesotho	59.2	68.3	9.1
Côte d'Ivoire	54.8	62.8	8.0
Nigeria	53.6	58.4	4.7

Source: 'The World at Six Billion', UN Development Programme, 12 October 1999

By 2010, life expectancy in many countries could be lower than at the beginning of the twentieth century, thus undermining virtually a century of developmental gains.[41]

In addition to decreasing average life expectancy, HIV/AIDS is expected to create up to 40m orphans in the years to come.[42] According to the UN definition, which includes children that have lost either their mother or both parents before the age of 15, the epidemic is already thought to have created 14m orphans, 11m of them in Sub-Saharan Africa. Table 8 (opposite) shows the numbers of orphans estimated to be living in selected African countries.

These children are exposed to the stigma of the illness, and are more vulnerable to malnutrition, illness, abuse and sexual exploitation.[43] Often, children are compelled to exchange sexual services in return for vital goods such as shelter, food, physical protection and money.[44] Even where this is not the case, and orphans are cared for by grandparents, there will be increasing dependence ratios between the old and the young.

Table 8: Number of AIDS Orphans, End-2000

Country	AIDS Orphans
Uganda	880,000
Nigeria	1,000,000
Ethiopia	990,000
Tanzania	810,000
Zimbabwe	780,000
Kenya	890,000
DRC	930,000
Zambia	570,000
South Africa	660,000
Côte d'Ivoire	420,000

Source: 'Report on the Global HIV/AIDS Epidemic', UNAIDS, July 2002

There are at least three ways in which strains on the social fabric and civil society of states with high prevalence rates could potentially foster social confrontation in future.

Attacks against people living with HIV/AIDS

One way in which HIV/AIDS might exacerbate social tensions is by provoking fears amongst the general population regarding those living with HIV. Around the globe, especially in places where the disease still carries a strong stigma, people living with HIV/AIDS face severe abuse, some of it violent.[45] In Colombia, left-wing guerrillas of the Revolutionary Armed Forces of Colombia (FARC) reportedly ordered 30,000 inhabitants of Vista Hermosa to take HIV tests, and forced those who tested positive out of their homes. The inhabitants of the region have been compelled to carry an identity card with the result of the test.[46] In Chennai, India, a young man was burned to death in the summer of 1998 by people who believed he was living with HIV.[47] In Nonthaburi, Thailand, both the general public and police personnel have attacked an AIDS relief centre.[48] In 1998, a South African woman died as a result of a beating she received by her neighbours in the outskirts of Durban, after she revealed on World AIDS Day that she was HIV-positive. She was also a volunteer with the National Association of People Living With HIV/AIDS (NAPWA) of South Africa. After receiving initial warnings not to disseminate any information about HIV, the woman was beaten to death with sticks and stones. Incidents such as these will not destabilise societies as a whole, but they do indicate the level of stigma surrounding HIV/AIDS. This stigma in turn is an immense obstacle to attempts to address the illness openly and publicly.

Social divisions

HIV/AIDS may also lead to unrest amongst people living with HIV. Richard Holbrooke has argued that AIDS 'will create a unique, new untouchable caste' that could provoke violence and civil strife.[49] The AIDS pandemic could thus also lead a growing number of people to become disengaged from their societies, and seek alternative and potentially violent ways of securing their existence. High HIV prevalence rates may combine with other factors to produce severe discontent amongst populations. In August 2001, hundreds of demonstrators and children orphaned by AIDS took to the streets of the Ethiopian capital Addis Ababa urging the government to do more to stop the spread of the epidemic.[50]

Depending on the numbers of people involved, discontent such as this could be a much more significant factor in contributing to political instability. Indeed, in some countries, if all those who are HIV-positive voted the same way, they could easily form a major force in national politics. Currently, the elite-driven nature of politics in the most-affected states and the social stigma attached to HIV/AIDS mean that many people are not willing to identify publicly with the illness. This may change, however; Robert Mattes, for instance, has expressed concern about what will happen if those not being cared for begin to resign from political processes, refuse to invest in their future, cease to pay bills and stop making financial contributions to public services.[51]

Youth crime and armed bands

HIV/AIDS could also prompt a growth in violent crime, contributing to increased social tension and, concomitantly, political instability. George Fidas of the NIC argues that 'once you know you have HIV ... you develop a short-term life span mentality, and you want to provide for your family, provide for your status and glory, whatever, in a shorter period of time, so that accentuates ... corruption'.[52] In Sierra Leone, members of the Revolutionary United Front are reported to have justified their violent actions by claiming that they were going to die of AIDS anyway.[53] There are historical precedents for disease causing a rise in crime rates, such as the plague epidemic in India between 1896 and 1914.[54] Martin Schönteich, of the Institute for Security Studies in South Africa, links the rise of HIV/AIDS with an exponentially increasing crime rate for the next five to 20 years.[55]

The large number of orphans that AIDS is likely to generate could become a serious problem. These orphans are vulnerable to exploitation and radicalisation, and might turn to crime and militia membership in order to maintain their existence in the face of inadequate support from their families and communities.[56] In the major towns of the Democratic Republic of Congo, thousands of children roaming the streets could end up in armed bands.[57] In South Africa, Ashraf Grimwood, of the National AIDS Coalition, argues that 'children orphaned by AIDS will have no role models in the future and they will resort to crime to survive'.[58] South Africa is particularly susceptible because of its high numbers of young people and the large wealth discrepancies within the country, making crime potentially more rewarding than elsewhere. Criminal bands and militias can also perform important psychological functions, such as providing members with surrogate father-figures and role models.[59] Militias and organised bands can thus provide an attractive combination of shelter, food and self-esteem for young people with unstable social backgrounds and few education and employment prospects.

This is part of a larger historical correlation between the outbreak of civil unrest and the presence of a large number of discontented young people. Based on his study of revolutionary violence, Teitelbaum has found that revolutions 'have historically occurred in societies that had a marked "youth bulge" – that is, a relatively high proportion of the population aged fifteen to twenty-five compared with the population age twenty-five and older'.[60] The illness cycle of HIV/AIDS could contribute to such a 'youth bulge' by causing a marked decrease in the number of older adults in relation to those between 15 and 25. There is evidence that this process is beginning in Zimbabwe, although it remains unclear to what extent HIV/AIDS is driving it.[61]

The impact of AIDS on political stability

It is tempting to conclude that the scale of the AIDS pandemic will culminate in serious political instability in the worst-affected states.

Indeed, some analysts warn unequivocally that states will become weakened to the point of collapse due to HIV/AIDS.[62] As with the previously-discussed impact of HIV/AIDS on the armed forces, however, the relationship between HIV/AIDS and possible state collapse is much more complex than is often suggested, and serious questions remain as to whether HIV/AIDS alone will induce such processes. In the past, epidemics like the plague destroyed social cohesion when mortality rates reached around 40%. In the case of cholera in nineteenth-century Europe, where mortality was around 15% of the population, such widespread breakdown did not occur.[63] Even the worst-affected countries are not yet experiencing such high mortality rates due to AIDS.

Nor are all of the worst-affected states similar in terms of the resources at their disposal to address HIV/AIDS. Botswana, for example, has one of the world's highest adult HIV prevalence rates, at over 35%. In a population of 1.5m, around 330,000 people are living with HIV. The country has taken a comparatively comprehensive approach to its response to the pandemic. In 2001, President Festus Mogae promised to provide drug therapies to all of Botswana's infected people. He is able to do so because Botswana also has what many other countries facing high HIV prevalence rates lack, namely resources. Botswana has prospered from diamond and cattle sales, accumulating over $7 billion in foreign reserves, and it has one of the most developed health care systems in the region.[64] The country is thus exceptional in that the need to address the epidemic has been recognised and acknowledged; the resources to tackle it are present; and the relatively small size of the population makes a solution feasible, at least in the short term. Important economic and environmental questions still remain about whether Botswana can sustain its level of wealth in the same way in the decades to come.

Those states most vulnerable to collapse because of HIV/AIDS will already be severely weakened by a variety of other factors, such as poverty, and will have been unstable for some time. HIV/AIDS thus might have a destabilising effect by hastening and exacerbating other processes that are conducive to state collapse.[65] In these states, HIV/AIDS poses serious new challenges to political stability. To date, little is known about how smaller effects multiplying and accumulating over the course of a decade or more affect a state's political stability. These kinds of implications are likely to be more difficult to discern, assess and predict. Societies have become more complex in the course of the twentieth century, and social expectations have changed. This makes it conceivable that smaller increases in the mortality rate than in the past could give rise to social dissolution.

Although the focus of this paper has been on countries where prevalence rates are highest, these new challenges to political stability should be of considerable concern to Western states. First, as already noted, delicate political constellations might be altered in the long run due to HIV/AIDS in regimes friendly to the West, or where the West has interests. Second, it may pose problems for countries that have traditionally made a large contribution to the maintenance of international peace and security in Africa, such as Nigeria and South Africa. Third, if in future HIV/AIDS contributes to instability, this might require costly and dangerous interventions which could result in members of the West's armed forces becoming HIV-positive.

A fourth reason why the weakening of state structures should be of concern to the West emerged particularly clearly on 11 September 2001. A marked decrease in state capacity also poses problems for the West in that it provides fertile ground from which terrorist and criminal networks can operate. This has led British Foreign Minister Jack Straw to argue that, in the twenty-first century, the real threat is no longer that of states with too much power, as was the case in the twentieth century, but states with too little. Straw argues that 'terrorists are strongest where states are weakest. Usama Bin Laden and the Al-Qa'ida network find safe havens in places – not just Afghanistan – where conflict, poverty, ethnic and racial tensions, exploitation, corruption, poor governance, malign interference from outside or just plain neglect have brought about the collapse of responsible government and civil society'.[66] While this overlooks the role played by 'stronger' states in training and harbouring many of these terrorists, it is also true that, where states have become weak, other groups such as warlords, criminal networks and terrorists can easily find harbour.

Finally, Western states could in future become directly affected by rising rates of HIV/AIDS. One of the greatest threats to civilians and armed forces operating and working abroad comes from infectious diseases, of which HIV/AIDS is one important example. People returning from overseas could introduce a new and potentially drug-resistant strain into their countries. There is consequently an inherent risk in letting the virus run unhindered in other areas of the world given its ability to mutate quickly. US scientists analysing the various strains of HIV are already observing that, in the conflict in the Democratic Republic of Congo, new versions are emerging. According to scientists at Los Alamos National Laboratory in New Mexico, 'something strange is going on in Congo. It's as if all the African HIV clades [subtypes] are mixing there, forming strange recombinants. We're seeing variants never seen before'.[67] Prior to the outbreak of conflict in the Congo, there was a fairly robust geographical distinction in the various subtypes of HIV, with types A and D predominating in the Lake Victoria region, and a comparatively newer subtype C, predominant in southern Africa, as well as in Ethiopia and the Horn. In West Africa, types A, G and D were the most prominent subtypes. With the advent of the conflict, however, Los Alamos scientist Bette Korber notes that 'recombination is happening so fast that we see the clade distinctions beginning to blur', with the emergence of new viruses that consist in part of different strains. Scientists are unsure what the long-term effect of this mixing will be, and whether it will lead to new or increased dangers. Irrespective of the DRC, researchers from the Center for Disease Control in Atlanta have begun to detect a new class of HIV that could trigger infection resistant to AZT (zidovudine) and possibly to stavudine.[68] In other words, the virus might not indefinitely remain under relative control in Western societies.

Conclusion

High prevalence rates of HIV/AIDS can exacerbate a variety of economic, political and social tensions. In so doing, HIV/AIDS also contributes to all three trajectories usually associated with processes of political instability and state collapse, and it is pushing developments further in this direction. In this sense, too, it has an important strategic dimension. In light of the differences between countries, and their varying levels of resources, we will only be able to determine how serious this impact will be on a country-by-country basis; research on this is in most cases lacking. Although it is possible to identify the key variables and trajectories, there is a clear need, as with the armed forces, for sustained and focused research on individual countries.

The second overall way in which HIV/AIDS is likely to have an important strategic dimension, both for those countries directly affected and for those with interests in these regions, is by way of the tensions that it intensifies within countries that are already struggling for resources and for stability. The significance of this will grow considerably in the years to come, as mortality rates increase, and will be felt in other areas of the globe as well. Most of the examples that have emerged to date relate to Africa, but the epidemic is also spreading in other areas. Although these regions may not experience the very high prevalence rates of Africa, they are nevertheless expected to see levels that are appreciably higher than in western European countries.

Yet, given the relatively long cycle of progression from HIV to AIDS, there is still an opportunity for concerted efforts to make medicines available to people living with HIV/AIDS. Indeed, there is an important difference between prevalence rates and mortality. In the case of HIV/AIDS, staggering prevalence rates of 30% or more of the adult population translate into a significantly smaller annual mortality rate, especially when measured as a percentage of the total population, rather than just the adult population. In South Africa, for example, the combined number of projected adult AIDS cases and deaths each year over the next decade is between 1.5% and 4% of the adult population.[69] These figures are clearly serious, and represent an immense humanitarian tragedy, especially because they will occur year after year. Yet they also point to a crisis that is, with sufficient resources and effort, still manageable, rather than one that is catastrophic in the full sense of being beyond hope. The most prudent strategy to avert state collapse would be to act now, before mortality rates increase still further. If such efforts are not forthcoming in the near future, state collapse cannot be ruled out.

Conclusion

If every age has its defining malady, then in those countries currently experiencing high HIV prevalence rates the present age will undoubtedly come to be characterised by AIDS. In these societies, virtually no aspect of social existence is untouched by this illness. The security sector is little different from any other sector of society which depends on healthy human beings to function effectively, and which is undermined by high morbidity and mortality rates. However, there are factors that make armed forces more prone to being affected by HIV/AIDS than civilian populations. Consequently, analysts must take more seriously the growing burden of widespread illnesses such as HIV/AIDS when surveying the contemporary strategic landscape. Within the conventional understanding of strategic analysis the growing AIDS pandemic gives rise to at least two important trajectories that will need to be researched closely in the years to come: first, the impact of the AIDS pandemic on the operational efficiency of armed forces in countries where prevalence rates are high, and the concomitant implications for international peacekeeping operations; and second, the extent to which HIV/AIDS contributes to political instability in states that are already weak, or that may become weakened in future due to a significant growth of the pandemic. There is nothing to prevent this general framework for thinking about the strategic dimensions of HIV/AIDS from also being applied to other illnesses, including ones that might emerge in the years to come. AIDS, after all, is not the only widespread illness currently ravaging the world, and tuberculosis and malaria are at least two other serious cases that also need to be analysed in greater detail and with due sensitivity to the particularities of the respective illnesses.

This paper has found that there is a clear and strategic dimension to the AIDS pandemic in the sense that it is raising important issues for the armed forces in many countries, and that it is posing considerable economic, political and social challenges to the most seriously-affected states. The AIDS pandemic thus already presents novel challenges, both for governments controlling the use of armed force in the international system, and for the militaries responsible for implementing any decision to deploy such force. This emerging strategic dimension also means that contemporary strategic experience is moving back in line with earlier historical experience. Prior to the twentieth century, it would not have surprised observers that diseases cost many more lives than armed conflicts, both amongst civilians and amongst the armed forces. It is only in the course of the twentieth century that this trend was reversed through advances in the ability to combat and eradicate certain diseases, and the simultaneous emergence of an industrial type of warfare that vastly increased the number of casualties resulting from armed conflicts. Today, HIV/AIDS and other widespread illnesses are beginning to reverse this trend.[1] The latter half of the twentieth century may well turn out to be a historical anomaly with regard to the interplay of disease and conflict, and strategic thinking must also evolve in a way that reflects these important changes.

Yet it is also necessary to begin thinking of HIV/AIDS in ways that do not characterise it exclusively as an overwhelming destabilising threat. As well as potentially further stigmatising people, a response based primarily on anxiety will only exacerbate the strategic dimension of HIV/AIDS. In the economic realm, for example, an overly pessimistic assessment can quickly turn into a self-fulfilling prophecy if investment in the economies of countries with high prevalence rates is reduced. In the social realm, eliciting a response of fear is also likely to increase the stigma attached to the illness; many of the social problems outlined in the previous chapters are not inherent, but are closely linked to the way in which the illness is perceived by citizens and policymakers. Finally, in the military realm an overly rash and drastic assessment of the impact of HIV/AIDS on the armed forces might increase the chance of strategic miscalculation. Precisely because the strategic challenges of HIV/AIDS are potentially very serious in the long run, a responsible, committed and reasonable response is required. For this reason, this paper has sought to make the case for a mature debate on the strategic dimension of HIV/AIDS – one which, while not ignoring this important dimension of the pandemic, also recognises the complexities surrounding this issue. The challenge of HIV/AIDS is certainly immense and serious, but in light of the long illness cycle there is still an important opportunity for joint responses focusing on the wider provision of medicines and the promotion of a more open culture surrounding the illness. The security sector could play a vital and responsible role in such responses.

In many ways, the most important variable is how individual governments and the international community respond to the global challenge of AIDS. This will depend on how political leaders engage with this issue, what resources they allocate to it and how they think about the illness. There are at least three reasons that speak in favour of responding now rather than later to the strategic dimension of the growing AIDS pandemic. First, and pending a viable cure and vaccine, it would be a very risky social and strategic experiment simply to let HIV/AIDS rage in strategically significant countries such as Russia, China and India. Second, the financial cost of addressing the pandemic now are likely to be much lower than if it culminates in more serious strategic risks in future. Third, the strategic dimension is only one, and perhaps not even the most important, aspect of the illness. One does not need to view this issue exclusively or even essentially as a strategic issue in order to recognise the profound social and humanitarian consequences this illness is having in many parts of the world. History is unlikely to judge kindly leaders and policymakers who refuse to address this issue, especially when resources and medicines are available and the pandemic is, in principle, manageable.

What, then, should the role of the security sector be in the response to the AIDS pandemic? Not all would agree that it should have a role at all: 'it is not quite clear', one strategist has noted, 'how military action can help stop the AIDS epidemic that is sweeping Africa and other parts of the world'.[2] On one level this is undoubtedly true; there cannot be a military solution to the global AIDS pandemic. Moreover, there are immense political and human-rights concerns associated with having the military sector alone take charge of the formulation and execution of the global response to HIV/AIDS.[3] Yet the opposite would also not seem viable. In light of the strategic dimensions of HIV/AIDS identified in this paper, any international response to the AIDS pandemic that operates in isolation from the security sector is also unlikely to prove successful in the long run. The AIDS pandemic cannot be successfully addressed in future if the important strategic dimension of the illness is not appreciated, and, by extension, if the security sector does not play a responsible role in this wider effort.

The security sector should pursue a two-fold strategy. First, and in relation to the specific impact of HIV/AIDS on the armed forces, militaries around the world should devote more funds, resources and effort to preventing the transmission of HIV/AIDS both within the armed forces, and between the armed forces and the civilian population. They will have to do this with due consideration for the human rights of individual soldiers, and with a concern for the human dimension of the illness. People living with the virus are not the enemy in the quest to address this issue, but will play a key part in future improvements. Consequently, they must also be included in these processes. Some armed forces have argued that people living with HIV should be excluded from the armed forces because they are not fit to function as soldiers, because the health of HIV-positive soldiers is compromised by the psychological and physical demands of serving in the armed forces, and because such people can become cognitively impaired while performing highly-skilled operations. These arguments are not currently backed by the weight of medical evidence.[4] Moreover, the time from initial infection to developing symptoms of AIDS is long, in some cases in excess of ten years. During this period a person can live without diseases or symptoms, with good health and normal functional capacity. HIV status alone is thus not an indicator of fitness to serve, and should not be used as a basis for excluding people living with HIV from the armed forces. Nor must HIV-positive people necessarily pose a risk to others, if they are encouraged to practice responsible sexual intercourse, and if basic blood-screening precautions recommended by the WHO are followed. Using soldiers as 'walking blood banks' for blood transfusion is medically unsafe irrespective of HIV, and should be discouraged.

A policy seeking to exclude people living with HIV might also have adverse effects. It is likely to clash with emerging legal and human-rights norms, especially the rights related to privacy, health, employment and non-discrimination.[5] This not only makes such policies ethically unjust, but also susceptible to legal challenge, as has already occurred in Namibia, Australia, Canada and India. With the exception of India, the courts upheld the challenge to such policies. Not only could such a policy culminate in expensive and potentially embarrassing high-profile court cases that damage civil-military relations, but it would also further undermine the security of these countries - much more so than keeping these people within the forces. Given that people living with HIV and who are not yet suffering from AIDS can usually carry out their duties for several years, the armed forces would be losing a considerable proportion of their manpower and expertise by excluding them, especially in the case of armed forces with high prevalence rates. Such a move would also mean that the armed forces would close themselves off from a considerable proportion of their conscription pools, as well as from those potential recruits who might refuse to join if they knew that this entailed a compulsory HIV test. Nor would such a policy address the issue of people who become HIV-positive whilst serving in the military. If the only HIV-positive people in the military became so whilst serving, this would reinforce the perception that the armed forces are a vector of the illness, and that serving in the military is a high-risk occupation. Excluding people living with HIV from the armed forces, in short, would be neither a just nor a strategically sound option.

Specifically, the armed forces in all regions of the world should ensure that they take the following steps to address the issue of HIV/AIDS within their ranks:

- implement and evaluate HIV/AIDS education programmes for members of the armed services that both discuss the illness in an open, serious and interactive manner, and that work to reduce the stigma attached to the illness;
- make voluntary and fully confidential testing available on a widespread basis, including counselling both before and after the test; this has proved more effective than compulsory testing in altering unsafe sexual behaviour, and also reduces the risks associated with false negative test results;
- make condoms of adequate standard widely and cheaply available within the armed forces, and encourage responsible sexual behaviour as part of the military ethos;

- implement just and humane procedures for those who are HIV-positive by allowing them to perform their duties for as long as possible where it is medically advisable for them to do so, and providing adequate care for them when they are no longer able to do so;
- re-evaluate which military practices are high risk with regard to HIV transmission and make amendments where possible;
- in those armed forces with advanced medical infrastructures, continue research for a viable and affordable AIDS vaccine and treat existing sexually-transmitted diseases;
- ensure blood safety in the armed forces by adopting and implementing adequate screening measures; and
- use active and demobilised soldiers as community HIV/AIDS educators, which not only generates employment for demobilising soldiers, but also raises their own awareness of HIV/AIDS and improves the image of the armed forces in the civilian population.

The military, with its unique organisational structure and captive audience, lends itself well to implementing many of these measures, which would allow it to take a prominent role in the quest to reduce the scale of the pandemic in the years to come. In this way, the security sector would work not only in its own interest, but would also be acting in the interest of good civil-military relations in the sense of reducing the transmission of HIV from the armed forces to the civilian population. Indeed, those few countries that have been able to reduce HIV prevalence are those where the military has been on board from an early point, and where the issue has been addressed in an open and humane fashion.

In addition to these specific measures, an effective strategy for the security sector would also incorporate a greater appreciation for the wider efforts being made to combat the pandemic. This is necessary because the root causes of the AIDS pandemic are located in a much broader set of economic, political and structural conditions that will have to be re-evaluated and partially alleviated if any attempt to tackle the spread of the pandemic is to be successful. These are aspects of the AIDS pandemic that the security sector is not ideally placed to address, and yet which nevertheless represent the broader context within which it operates. Rather, the security sector would do well to recognise the convergence of interest with regards to addressing the global AIDS pandemic, and be broadly supportive of this wider endeavour. This would certainly be prudent in light of the possible long-term impact of HIV/AIDS on political stability, because the armed forces constitute a high-risk group with regards to HIV, and because of the overwhelming humanitarian dimension of the illness. Any reduction in overall prevalence rates would also alleviate the problems increasingly confronted by armed forces with regards to HIV/AIDS. It is thus also in the interest of armed forces to endorse governmental contributions to local and international efforts to reduce the transmission of HIV/AIDS such as the Global Fund to Fight AIDS, Tuberculosis & Malaria. At the same time, the root causes of the pandemic – which clearly extend far beyond the virus itself - will not be overcome without assistance from the international community, which similarly needs to invest much more resources in such efforts. Ideally, there would be a sustained dialogue at the local, regional and international levels to discern the best strategies for the regions affected, and in order to ensure that efforts are compatible with local practices and expectations.

Finally, strategic analysts must also adapt to the changes that the world is undergoing due to the AIDS pandemic. We currently know much less about the long-term strategic implications of HIV/AIDS than we think we do – too little, in fact – and there is a clear need for more country-specific research on the strategic implications of HIV/AIDS if national and international public policy is to be made on an informed basis in the years to come. HIV/AIDS additionally signals a need to rethink and amend the more conventional notion of strategy. The military understanding of strategy did not emerge in a historical vacuum, but was itself a response to the social reality of the twentieth century, during which the two world wars inflicted high degrees of human suffering and hardship on entire societies, during which the Cold War threatened to incur even more, and during which the significance of lethal infectious diseases declined in the Western world. HIV/AIDS is already having social ramifications not dissimilar to those traditionally associated with the effects of armed conflicts. Like many previous wars, HIV/AIDS is beginning to erode the social, economic, political and demographic fabric of societies faced with high prevalence rates.

For Clausewitz, war was famously the continuation of politics by other means. In light of the tragic humanitarian implications of AIDS and the millions of lives wagered, it might today be tempting to adapt this dictum and suggest that the conduct of international politics is increasingly the continuation of a silent war by other means. Perhaps this will only be remedied in the twenty-first century if strategy itself becomes at least partially the continuation of medicine by other means. This is the ultimate challenge for strategy in the age of AIDS.

Notes

Introduction

1. John Keegan, *War and Our World: The Reith Lectures 1998* (London: Hutchinson, 1998), pp. 1, 17.
2. HIV stands for Human Immunodeficiency Virus, AIDS for Acquired Immunodeficiency Syndrome.
3. United Nations Press Release SC/6781, 10 January 2000.
4. According to UNAIDS, there have been cases in the Great Lakes region of Africa of women being raped by soldiers 'with the stated intent of infecting them with HIV'. 'UN Security Council Meeting on HIV/AIDS in Africa: Briefing Pack', UNAIDS, 10 January 2000, p. 7.
5. For one notable exception, see Marcella David, 'Rubber Helmets: The Certain Pitfalls of Marshalling Security Council Resources To Combat AIDS in Africa', *Human Rights Quarterly*, vol. 23, no. 3, 2001, pp. 560-82.
6. J. Stephen Morrison, 'HIV/AIDS', in *A Review of US Africa Policy*, Draft Discussion Document for Presentation at the Woodrow Wilson Center Conference, 'The Future of US Africa Policy', Center for Strategic and International Studies, Washington DC, December 2000, pp. 30-31. See also *AIDS and Violent Conflict in Africa*, United States Institute of Peace Special Report, 15 October 2001, p. 1.

Chapter 1

1. Ralph H. Major, *War and Disease* (London: Hutchison, 1941), p. 16.
2. *Ibid.*, p. 185; William H. McNeill, *Plagues and Peoples* (Toronto: Doubleday, 1989), p. 10.
3. Hans Zinsser, *Rats, Lice, and History* (London: George Routledge, 1937), p. 153.
4. Major, *War and Disease*, pp. 66-67.
5. *Ibid.*, p. 68.
6. Lester Brown, Gary Gardner and Brian Halweil, *Beyond Malthus: Nineteen Dimensions of the Population Challenge* (New York: W. W. Norton, 1999), p. 122.
7. Ann Hwang, 'AIDS Over Asia: AIDS Has Arrived in India and China', *The Guardian*, 16 January 2001.
8. John Gittings, 'War on Prejudice as China Awakes to HIV Nightmare', *ibid.*, 3 November 2000.
9. 'Report on the Global HIV/AIDS Epidemic', UNAIDS, July 2002.
10. *Ibid.*
11. 'The Global Strategy Framework on HIV/AIDS', UNAIDS, June 2001, p. 3.
12. 'AIDS and the Military', UNAIDS, May 1998, p. 2.

13 Lindy Heinecken, 'AIDS: The New Security Frontier', *Conflict Trends*, vol. 3, no. 4, 2000, www.accord.org.za.

14 Len Curran and Michael Munywoki, 'HIV/AIDS and Uniformed Services: Stocktaking of Activities in Kenya, Tanzania and Uganda', UNAIDS, August 2002, p. 10.

15 Jean Le May, 'More than Half of South Africa's Army "May have HIV"', *The Independent*, 15 July 2002.

16 Paul Kirk, 'Sixty Percent of Army May Be HIV-Positive', *The Mail and Guardian*, 31 March 2000; 'Up to 70% of South African Army Infected', UN Wire, 5 April 2000.

17 *Ibid*.

18 *Ibid*.

19 'HIV-AIDS Rife in Namibia Defence Forces', *Panafrican News Agency*, 16 February 2001.

20 James Astill, 'War Injects AIDS into Sierra Leone: Two out of Three Soldiers Could Be Infected with the Virus, According to a United Nations Report', *The Guardian*, 21 May 2001.

21 According to the Civil-Military Alliance to Combat HIV and AIDS based in Switzerland, a survey of 198 members of the Umbutfo Swaziland Defence Force seeking treatment for other sexually-transmitted diseases in early 1997 indicated that 42% were HIV-positive, while HIV prevalence in the military was around 16% in Côte d'Ivoire in 1994 (Factsheet: 'HIV Prevalence in the Military'). According to the US Census Bureau, in 1993 military prevalence rates in Cameroon were reported to be 6.2%, while studies of 11 garrisons and ten camps carried out in Cameroon in 1996 indicated prevalence rates of 12% and 14.7% respectively. A study of 257 military personnel carried out in N'Djamena, Chad, between January and March 1995 indicated a prevalence rate of 10.1%, while a 1996 study of army personnel in the Central African Republic showed a prevalence rate of 13.9%. A study of military personnel in Tanzania in 1994 indicated a prevalence rate of 12.9%, while studies of military recruits in 1994-97 in Uganda indicate a prevalence rate of 25-29%, depending on the age group. 'HIV/AIDS Surveillance Database', Population Division, International Programs Center, Washington DC, June 2000.

22 Roxanne Bazergan, 'UN Peacekeepers and HIV/AIDS', *World Today*, vol. 57, no. 5, May 2001, p. 7.

23 Leo Dobbs, 'AIDS Looms Large over Cambodian Military, Police', *Reuters*, 5 October 1995.

24 'HIV/AIDS Surveillance Database', US Census Bureau.

25 Stuart Kingma, Director of the Civil-Military Alliance to Combat HIV and AIDS, cited in *AIDS and Men - Old Problem, New Angle* (London: Panos Institute, 1998).

26 K. E. Nelson *et al.*, 'Changes in Sexual Behavior and a Decline in HIV Infection among Young Men in Thailand', *New England Journal of Medicine*, vol. 335, 1 August 1996, pp. 297-303.

27 '4.5 Percent of Recruits Test Positive in Vietnam Province', *Associated Press*, 7 January 2002; 'HIV/AIDS Surveillance Database', US Census Bureau.

28 'Sharp Rise in Number of HIV-Positive Russian Troops: Report', *Agence France-Presse*, 5 October 2000.

29 Uncas Fernandez, 'Soaring HIV Infection Rate, Denial Have Brazil's Military under the Gun', *Agence France-Presse*, 3 December 1996.

30 Johanna Mendelson Forman and Manuel Carballo, 'A Policy Critique of HIV/AIDS and Demobilisation', *Conflict, Security and Development*, vol. 1, no. 2, p. 78.

31 Rodger Yeager, 'AIDS Brief: Military Populations', Civil-Military Alliance to Combat HIV and AIDS.

32 Rodger Yeager and Donna Ruscavage, 'HIV Prevention and Behavior Change in International Military Populations', CERTI Crisis and Transition Tool Kit, September 2000.

33 'AIDS and the Military', p. 2.

34 *Ibid.*, p. 3.

35 *Ibid.*

36 'AIDS and the Military', UNAIDS, p. 5.

37 Naval Medical Surveillance Report, vol. 4, no. 2, April-June 2001, p. 5.

38 *Ibid.*, p. 12.

Chapter 2

1 Kingma, 'AIDS Prevention in Military Populations - Learning the Lessons of History', *International AIDS Society Newsletter*, no. 4, March 1996, cited in Manuel Carballo, Carolyn Mansfield and Michaela Prokop, 'Demobilization and Its Implications for HIV/AIDS', CERTI Crisis and Transition Tool Kit, October 2000.

2 Heinecken, 'AIDS: The New Security Frontier'.

3 Major, *War and Disease*, p. 112.

4 Astill, 'War Injects AIDS into Sierra Leone'.

5 Lindy Heinecken, 'Living in Terror: The Looming Security Threat to Southern Africa', *African Security Review*, vol. 10, no. 4, 2001, pp. 11-12.

6 Lindy Heinecken, 'Strategic Implications of HIV/AIDS in South Africa', *Conflict, Security and Development*, vol 1, no. 1, 2001, p. 110.

7 'Global HIV/AIDS: A Strategy for US Leadership', A Consensus Report of the Center for Strategic and International Studies Working Group on Global HIV/AIDS, Washington DC, 1994, p. 3.

8 'HIV-AIDS Rife In Namibia Defence Forces'.

9 Greg Mills, 'AIDS and the South African Military: Timeworn Cliché or Timebomb?', Occasional Paper, Konrad Adenauer Foundation (KAF), 2000.

10 See Robert Shell, 'Trojan Horses: HIV/AIDS and Military Bases in Southern Africa', unpublished paper, 2000, p. 1.

11 J. Ntarindawa, 'Armed Forces HIV/AIDS Control Strategies and Activities', Ministry of Defence, Republic of Rwanda, January 1999, cited in Forman and Caballo, 'A Policy Critique of HIV/AIDS', p. 76.

12 *Newsletter of the Civil-Military Alliance to Combat HIV and AIDS*, vol. 4, no. 1, January 1998, p. 2.

13 Cynthia Enloe, *Bananas, Beaches and Bases* (Berkley, CA: University of California Press, 1990), pp. 88-89.

14 Quoted in 'AIDS and the Military', UNAIDS, p. 7.

15 'Deputy Minister of Defence Sounds Warning Against HIV/AIDS', *Namibian Government News*, 11 July 2001; Ntarindwa, 'Armed Forces HIV/AIDS Control Strategies and Activities'.

16 Heinecken, 'Strategic Implications of HIV/AIDS', p. 110.

17 'South Africa: Defence Force to Create HIV Database', *SAPA News Agency*, 1 March 2001.

18 John B. Chittick, *The Coming Wave: HIV/AIDS in Vietnam*, self-published, 1996, Chapter 2.

19 *Ibid.*

20 K. Ireland, 'Report of Training Programme on Community Based AIDS Prevention Strategies', Asian Center for Population and Community Development, Bangkok, 17-28 June 1991, p. 13, cited in Chittick, *The Coming Wave*, Chapter 2.

21 *Ibid.*

22 *Ibid.* In Namibia, by contrast, a judge ruled on 10 May 2000 that HIV infection alone does not constitute legitimate grounds for barring an applicant.

23 Chittick, *The Coming Wave*, Chapter 2.

24 Joe Cochrane, 'HIV/AIDS Now Cambodian Military's Only Enemy', *Deutsche Presse-Agentur*, 31 March 1999.

25 *Ibid*.

26 *Ibid*.

27 'China Begins HIV/AIDS Tests for Military Recruits', *Agence France-Presse*, 25 October 2001.

28 Peter W. Singer, 'AIDS and International Security', *Survival*, vol. 44, no. 1, Spring 2002, pp. 145-46.

29 *World Military Expenditures and Arms Transfers 1999-2000* (Washington DC: US Department of State, Bureau of Verification and Compliance, October 2001), p. 5.

30 Paul Beaver, comments on *Voice of America*, 3 May 2000.

31 Chittick, *The Coming Wave*, Chapter 2.

32 *Ibid*.

33 Astill, 'War Injects AIDS into Sierra Leone'.

34 Chris Allen, 'Warfare, Endemic Violence and State Collapse in Africa', *Review of African Political Economy*, no. 81, 1999, p. 371.

35 Lanre Babalola, 'ECOMOG Soldiers Storm Synagogue for HIV/AIDS Treatment', *PM News* (Lagos), 1 December 2001.

Chapter 3

1 See, for example, Rodger Yeager, 'AIDS Briefs: Military Populations', Civil-Military Alliance to Combat HIV and AIDS.

2 Richard Holbrooke, comments on *Voice of America*, 8 June 2000.

3 Mark Schoofs, 'A New Kind of Crisis: The Security Council Declares AIDS in Africa a Threat to World Stability', *The Village Voice*, 12-18 January 2000.

4 Astill, 'War Injects AIDS into Sierra Leone'.

5 *UN Peacekeeping: United Nations Faces Challenges in Responding to the Impact of HIV/AIDS on Peacekeeping Operations* (Washington DC: US General Accounting Office, December 2001), p. 8.

6 Jia Kangbai, 'one out of ten of city dwellers tested HIV positive', *The Progress*, 13 August, 2001.

7 Erich Follath, 'Robin Hood und die Multis', *Der Spiegel*, no. 14, 2001, p. 158.

8 Bazergan, 'UN Peacekeepers and HIV/AIDS', p. 7.

9 Remarks by Ambassador Richard C. Holbrooke, United States Permanent Representative to the United Nations, on Implementation of Resolution 1308 on AIDS, at the Security Council, 22 December 2000.

10 Carolyn Nordstrom, 'Behind the Lines', *New Routes*, vol. 2, no. 1, 1997.

11 UN Peacekeeping, p. 24.

12 A. Adefolalu, 'HIV/AIDS as an Occupational Hazard to Soldiers - ECOMOG Experience', paper presented at the Third All African Congress of Armed Forces and Police Medical Services, Pretoria, 24-28 October 1999, cited in Stuart Kingma and Rodger Yeager, 'A Civil-Military Alliance Response to the HIV/AIDS Epidemic in Nigeria', concept paper prepared for the US Agency for International Development, February 2000.

13 Maggie Farley, 'UN Seeks To Curb Role in Spread of AIDS Health: World Organization Wages Campaign To Curtail International Peacekeepers' Involvement in Transmission of the Disease', *Los Angeles Times*, 7 January 2000.

14 'US International Strategy on HIV/AIDS'.

15 'Obasanjo Warns Soldiers against Unprotected Sex', *Agence France-Presse*, 19 May 2000.

16 Omololu Falobi, 'Nigerian

Government Admits HIV Infection Among ECOMOG Soldiers', AF-AIDS, 4 January 2000.

[17] Heinecken, 'AIDS: The New Security Frontier'.

[18] Farley, 'UN Seeks To Curb Role'.

[19] 'Indian Soldiers Returning From UN Duty in Cambodia Test HIV Positive', *United Press International*, 5 September 1993; *UN Peacekeeping*, p. 10.

[20] Joe Lauria, 'UN Expected To OK Condom-a-Day Funds: $2M Yearly Bill Likely for Troops', *Boston Globe*, 22 March 2000, cited in Marie-France Guimond, Noah S. Philip and Usman Sheikh, 'Health Concerns of Peacekeeping: A Survey of the Current Situation', 13 July 2001, www.jha.ac/articles/a067.htm.

[21] Chris Beyrer, *War in the Blood: Sex, Politics and AIDS in Southeast Asia* (New York: Zed Books, 1998), pp. 64-65.

[22] 'The Future Strategic Context for Defence', UK Ministry of Defence, 7 February 2001, paragraph 19.

[23] Mills, 'AIDS and the South African Military', p. 70.

[24] *Ibid*.

[25] 'Infected Troops Spread a Scourge Worse Than War', *San Jose Mercury News*, 8 April 2001, cited in 'HIV/AIDS as a Security Issue', International Crisis Group, 19 June 2001, p. ii.

[26] Heinecken, 'Strategic Implications of HIV/AIDS', p. 111.

[27] 'Sexual Behavior of Soldiers Must Change: SANDF', *South African Press Association*, 2 August 2001.

[28] Bazergan, 'UN Peacekeepers and HIV/AIDS', p. 6.

[29] 'Official Concern Over Sex Case and HIV/AIDS', *UN Integrated Regional Information Network*, 1 September 2001.

[30] Simon Robinson, 'Battle Ahead', *Time*, 16 July 2001.

[31] Forman and Carballo, 'A Policy Critique of HIV/AIDS and Demobilisation', p. 77.

[32] 'HIV/AIDS as a Security Issue', p. 19.

[33] 'Eritrean Troops, UN Peacekeepers End AIDS Prevention Training', *Agence France-Presse*, 30 July 2001.

[34] Thalif Deen, 'UN Focuses on Links Between AIDS and Peacekeeping', *Inter Press Service*, 17 July 2000; *UN Peacekeeping*, p. 11.

[35] Yeager, 'AIDS Briefs: Military Populations'.

[36] *UN Peacekeeping*, United States General Accounting Office, p. 3.

[37] Schoofs, 'A New Kind of Crisis'.

[38] Michelle Sieff, 'HIV/AIDS: Under Siege', *World Today*, May 2001, p. 5.

Chapter 4

[1] Barton Gellman, 'The Belated Global Response to AIDS in Africa', *Washington Post*, 5 July 2000.

[2] 'AIDS Epidemic Update', UNAIDS, December 2001, p. 18.

[3] Zinsser, *Rats, Lice and History*, p. 128.

[4] *Ibid.*, p. 129.

[5] Samantha Willan, 'A Concept Paper: Considering the Impact of HIV/AIDS on Democratic Governance and Vice Versa', unpublished paper, Health Economics & HIV/AIDS Research Division, University of Natal, June 2000, p. 9.

[6] I. William Zartman, 'Introduction: Posing the Problem of State Collapse', in Zartman (ed.), *Collapsed States: The Disintegration and Restoration of Legitimate Authority* (Boulder, CO: Lynne Rienner, 1995), p. 2.

[7] Chris Allen, 'Ending Endemic Violence: Limits to Conflict Resolution in Africa', *Review of African Political Economy*, vol. 26, no. 81, September 1999, pp. 318-19.

[8] 'HIV/AIDS Hitting the Armed Forces in Africa', *Panafrican News Agency*, 9 July 2001.

[9] Kofi Annan, 'Review of the Problem of Human Immunodeficiency Virus/Acquired Immunodeficiency Syndrome in All Its Aspects', A/55/779,

16 February 2001.

10 'HIV/AIDS: The Impact on Social and Economic Development', Third Report of the Select Committee on International Development, House of Commons, London, 29 March 2001, Section 2, § 113.

11 'Report on the Global HIV/AIDS Epidemic', UNAIDS, June 2000, p. 31.

12 Henri E Cauvin, 'Zimbabwe Fund for AIDS Patients is Frozen in Bureaucracy', *New York Times*, 19 August 2001.

13 'Global Trends 2015: A Dialogue About the Future With Nongovernment Experts', report of the National Intelligence Council, December 2000.

14 Annan, 'Review of the Problem', p. 8.

15 *Ibid.*, p. 9.

16 'Macroeconomics and Health: Investing in Health for Economic Development', Report of the Commission on Macroeconomics and Health, WHO, 2001, pp. 31-32.

17 Solomon R. Benatar, 'South Africa's Transition in a Globalizing World: HIV/AIDS as a Window and a Mirror', *International Affairs*, vol. 77, no. 2, 2001, p. 365.

18 'Cambodian Opposition Blasts Defence-dominated National Budget', *Agence France-Presse*, 13 December 1999.

19 'Situation Analysis: South Africa', US Agency for International Development, Washington DC, 2001.

20 Rodger Yeager and Stuart Kingma, 'HIV/AIDS Destabilising National Security and the Multi-National Response', *International Review of the Armed Forces Medical Services*, vol. 74, no. 3, 2001, pp. 3-12.

21 Markus Haacker, 'The Economic Consequences of HIV/AIDS in Southern Africa', IMF Working Paper WP/02/38, February 2002, pp. 34-35.

22 'Tanzania: AIDS Cause Nearly Half Women's Deaths In Dar', *TOMRIC News Agency* (Dar es Salaam), 24 April 2000.

23 'NamWater Counts the Costs of AIDS', *IRIN HIV/AIDS Weekly Issue*, no. 37, 27 July 2001, cited in Pieter Fourie and Martin Schönteich, 'The Impact of HIV/AIDS on Human Security in South and Southern Africa', paper presented at the ECPR Conference, Canterbury, 8-10 September 2001, p. 13.

24 'HIV/AIDS: The Impact on Social and Economic Development', Select Committee on International Development, Section 2, §116.

25 Raphael Tenthani, 'SADC Police Chiefs Warned To Regard AIDS as Security Issue', *Panafrican News Agency*, 31 July 2000. For Uganda, see 'HIV/AIDS Depleting Police Force, Says IG', *New Vision* (Kampala), 2 January 2002.

26 'AIDS Accounts for 75 Per Cent of Police Officers Deaths', *The Nation* (Nairobi), 27 November 2000; Sheikh Chifuwe, 'HIV/AIDS Devastates Police Service', *The Post* (Lusaka), 18 July 2001.

27 Donald G. McNeil Jr., 'AIDS Stalking Africa's Struggling Economies', *New York Times*, 15 November 1998.

28 A. Shaw, 'Under the Shadow of the Big Kill', *Globe and Mail*, 1 June 1996, cited in Andrew T. Price-Smith, *The Health of Nations: Infectious Disease, Environmental Change, and Their Effects on National Security and Development* (Cambridge, MA: MIT Press, 2001), p. 14; 'Six Ministers HIV-positive', *Financial Gazette*, 22 November 2001.

29 Comment by an audience member on a panel: 'HIV and Demobilization - The New Challenge to Theory and Practice', Demobilization Workshop, Nairobi, Kenya, 20 March 2001.

30 'Contagion and Conflict: Health as a Global Security Challenge',

Report of the Chemical and Biological Arms Control Institute and the CSIS International Security Program, Washington DC, January 2000, p. 29.

31 'Zambia Seeks HIV Test for Presidential Candidates', *Associated Press*, 2 November 2001.

32 Randy Cheek, 'Playing God with HIV: Rationing HIV Treatment in Southern Africa', *African Security Review*, vol. 10, no. 4, 2001, p. 20.

33 *Ibid.*, pp. 25-26.

34 Cecil Johnson, 'Broken British, US Promises Fuelled Land Protests In Zimbabwe', *St Paul Pioneer Press*, 1 May 2000. See also Heinecken, 'Strategic Implications of HIV/AIDS', p. 113.

35 Patrick Chabal and Jean-Pascal Daloz, *Africa Works: Disorder as a Political Instrument* (London: Villiers, 1999), p. xviii.

36 'HIV/AIDS: The Impact on Social and Economic Development', Select Committee on International Development, Section 2, §120.

37 *Ibid.*, §115.

38 'HIV/AIDS as a Security Issue', p. 16.

39 Annan, 'Review of the Problem of Human Immunodeficiency Virus', p. 8.

40 'The Global Infectious Disease Threat and Its Implications for the United States', report of the National Intelligence Council, NIE 99-17D, January 2000.

41 David Gordon, remarks at United States Institute for Peace Current Issues Briefing Panel 'Plague Upon Plague: AIDS and Violent Conflict in Africa', Washington DC, 8 May 2001.

42 'Global Trends 2015: A Dialogue About the Future With Nongovernment Experts'.

43 Annan, 'Review of the Problem', p. 9.

44 Ulf Kristoffersson, 'HIV/AIDS as a Human Security Issue: A Gender Perspective', paper presented at the expert group meeting on 'The HIV/AIDS Pandemic and Its Gender Implications', Windhoek, Namibia, 13-17 November 2000.

45 'Global HIV/AIDS: A Strategy for US Leadership', p. 7.

46 Martin Hodgson, 'Rebels Expel HIV Victims from Homes', *The Guardian*, 23 October 2001; and Juan Pablo Toro, 'Colombian Rebels Forcing AIDS Tests', *Associated Press*, 13 October 2001.

47 Sandra Thurman, 'Joining To Fight HIV and AIDS', *Washington Quarterly*, vol. 24, no. 1, Winter 2001, p. 194.

48 Chittick, *The Coming Wave*, Chapter 2.

49 Schoofs, 'A New Kind of Crisis'.

50 'AIDS Orphans Demonstrate', *UN Integrated Regional Information Network*, 6 August 2001.

51 Robert Mattes, cited in Willan, 'A Concept Paper', p. 11.

52 George Fidas, 'Infectious Disease and Global Security', presentation at the 'International Disease Surveillance and Global Security' Conference, Stanford University, Stanford, CA, 11 May 2001.

53 Paul Richards, 'Hurry, We are All Dying of AIDS: Linking Cultural and Agro-Technological Responses to the Challenge of Living with AIDS in Africa', unpublished paper, University of Wageningen, 1999, cited in Alex de Waal, 'How Will HIV/AIDS Transform African Governance?', unpublished paper, London 2002.

54 Rajnarayan Chandavarkar, 'Plague Panic and Epidemic Politics in India, 1896-1914', in Terence Ranger and Paul Slack, *Epidemics and Ideas: Essays on the Historical Perception of Pestilence* (Cambridge: Cambridge University Press, 1992), pp. 232-33.

55 Martin Schönteich, 'Age and AIDS: South Africa's Crime Time Bomb?', *African Security Review*, vol. 8, no. 4, 1999, cited in Robert Shell, 'Halfway to the Holocaust: The Economic, Demographic and Social Implications of the AIDS

Pandemic to the Year 2010 in the Southern African Region', in Michael Lange (ed.), *HIV/AIDS: A Threat to the African Renaissance?*, pp. 18-19.

⁵⁶ Jordan S. Kassalow, 'Why Health Is Important to US Foreign Policy', paper prepared for the Council on Foreign Relations, New York and Washington DC, April 2001, www.cfr.org.

⁵⁷ 'No End in Sight: The Human Tragedy of the Conflict in the Democratic Republic of Congo', Oxfam International (London), 6 August 2001.

⁵⁸ M. M. Mackay, 'AIDS Will Spur on Crime, Say Experts', *Saturday Argus*, 9 January 1999, cited in Martin Schönteich, 'The Impact of HIV/AIDS on South Africa's Internal Security', paper presented at the First Annual Conference of the South African Association of Public Administration and Management in Pretoria, 23 November 2000.

⁵⁹ Judith Large, 'Disintegration Conflicts and the Restructuring of Masculinity', *Gender and Development*, vol. 5, no. 2, June 1997, pp. 23-30.

⁶⁰ Cited in Jennifer Leaning and Sam Arie, 'Human Security in Crisis and Transition: A Background Document of Definition and Application', CERTI Crisis and Transition Tool Kit, September 2000.

⁶¹ 'Another Nail in Zimbabwe's Coffin', *Africa News Service*, 5 December 2000, cited in Heinecken, 'Strategic Implications of HIV/AIDS', p. 113.

⁶² Singer, 'AIDS and International Security', p. 146.

⁶³ See Richard Evans, 'Epidemics and Revolutions: Cholera in Nineteenth-century Europe', in Ranger and Slack, *Epidemics and Ideas*, p. 170.

⁶⁴ Tom Masland, 'Botswana's Hope', *Newsweek*, 11 June 2001, p. 81.

⁶⁵ Price-Smith, *The Health of Nations*, p. 121.

⁶⁶ 'Order Out of Chaos: The Future of Afghanistan', Speech by UK Foreign Secretary Jack Straw at IISS, London, 22 October 2001.

⁶⁷ Laurie Garrett, 'Allies of AIDS: Among Warring Factions in Congo, Disease Is Mutating', *Newsday*, 9 July 2000.

⁶⁸ 'New HIV Subtype May Be Tougher to Treat: CDC', *Reuters Health*, 7 November 2001.

⁶⁹ See Alan Whiteside and Clem Sunter, *AIDS: The Challenge for South Africa* (Cape Town: Human & Rousseau and Tafelberg, 2000), pp. 68-89.

Conclusion

¹ Harriet Hentges, remarks at the United States Institute for Peace Current Issues Briefing Panel 'Plague Upon Plague: AIDS and Violent Conflict in Africa'.

² James J. Wirtz, 'A New Agenda for Security and Strategy', in John Baylis *et al.* (eds), *Strategy in the Contemporary World: An Introduction to Strategic Studies* (Oxford: Oxford University Press, 2002), p. 311.

³ See Barry Buzan, Ole Wæver and Jaap de Wilde, *Security: A New Framework for Analysis* (Boulder, CO: Lynne Rienner, 1998).

⁴ See Eric A. Feldman, 'United Nations Peacekeeping Operations and Mandatory HIV Testing', Institution for Social and Policy Studies, Yale University, August 2001. See also UNAIDS, 'Report of the UNAIDS Expert Panel on HIV Testing in United Nations Peacekeeping Operations', Bangkok, 28-30 November 2001, p. 9.

⁵ See, for example, 'HIV Testing of UN Peacekeeping Forces: Legal and Human Rights Issues', *Canadian HIV/AIDS Legal Network*, 9 September 2001.